CONSUMER HEALTH:

Products and Services

CONSUMER HEALTH:

Products and Services

JESSIE HELEN HAAG, Ed.D., F.R.S.H.
Professor, Health Education
The University of Texas at Austin

LEA & FEBIGER *Philadelphia* • *1976*

Library of Congress Cataloging in Publication Data

Haag, Jessie Helen.
    Consumer health: products and services.

    Bibliography:
    1. Medical care—United States. 2. Public health personnel—United States.
3. Quacks and quackery—United States. 4. Consumer education—United States.
I. Title. [DNLM: 1. Chiropractic—Popular works. 2. Diet fads—Popular works. 3.
Insurance, Health—Popular works. 3. Quackery—Popular works. 4. Therapeutic
cults—Popular works. WZ310 Hlllа 1976]
RA445.H2   362.1'0973   74-6033
ISBN 0-8121 0562-1

Published in Great Britain by Henry Kimpton Publishers, London

PRINTED IN THE UNITED STATES OF AMERICA

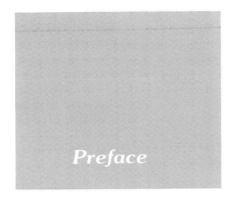

Preface

ONE of the content areas of school health education is consumer health. This content area may be defined as topics dealing with a wise selection of health products and services, agencies concerned with the control of these products and services, evaluation of quackery and health misconceptions, health careers, and health insurance.

Consumer health has grown to be one of the most popular and meaningful content areas of school health education. This text will provide information for the consumer to make wise decisions as to purchases of health products and services.

This text is intended for students in health education courses; students in nursing, medicine, and dentistry; and for professionals in allied health fields. Also, it may serve as a reference for elementary and secondary school teachers of health education, social studies, and home economics and for consumer protection agencies, insurance companies, and governmental regulatory agencies.

Austin, Texas   Jessie Helen Haag

Contents

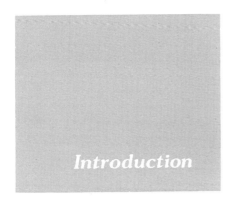

Introduction

TODAY'S consumer is bombarded with all types of advertising of health products and services. Some examples of health products are toothpastes, deodorants, antiperspirants, vitamin pills, cereals, remedies for indigestion, weight reduction devices, cures for arthritis, pills to increase sexual potency, and organic foods. Services advertised come from food faddists, mystical leaders of the occult, mechanotherapists, and psychoquacks. The cost of advertising these products and services exceeds $6 billion a year, not to mention the costs of the advertised items. The uninformed consumer believes he can buy a long life free of disease or disability.

The need for consumer health education is apparent from the prevalence of self-medication, the ignorance of rudimentary health facts, the widespread acceptance of quackery and the occult, and inadequate health insurance. Lack of information about health care, over-the-counter drugs, arthritis cures, and weight reduction devices is not uncommon.

Rising costs of medical care have forced many persons to indulge in self-medication or to postpone needed care. It has been estimated that the American public spends 148 percent more on health care than it did ten years ago. Costs of hospital care have increased 248 percent, physicians' services, 144 percent, and medicines and health appliances, 93 percent. Dental care has also increased in cost. Today's parents with a child under the care of an orthodontist may expect a costly dental bill.

Nationally televised health tests, polls by nationally known pollsters, and other studies have revealed the lack of valid health information of the American public. The National Health Test quizzed the public by television on rudimentary health facts and found generally poor health knowledge. The Harris organization found that 30 percent of the adults polled could not name one warning signal of cancer and 50 percent did not know one possible sign of a heart attack.

Americans spend more than $2 billion a year on quackery. Of that amount, at least $400 million is spent on worthless cures for arthritis, $50 million on cancer cures, and from $2 billion to $10 billion on weight-reducing devices. New types of quackery emerge each day because of the gullibility of the American public. The occult has boomed into a $200 million a year business with gurus, swamis, cultists, and witches who propound cures for every type of human disease and defect.

Fortunately, more Americans under and over 65 years of age have some type of health insurance. Medicare has provided hospital care to some 20 million persons. From 1961 to 1971, individual and family health insurance policies grew 96 percent. Insurance companies paid $9 billion in group health insurance benefits in 1971, three times more than in 1961. However, 17 million Americans under 65 years of age have no health insurance. At least one half have no insurance to pay physicians' bills outside a hospital and no health insurance for surgery. Many families, although "insured," could be wiped out financially because of a serious, prolonged illness.

In this last quarter of the twentieth century, the American consumer needs to make a wise selection of health products and services, and use the consumer protection agencies at the local, state, and federal levels. Consumer health education can be an important step toward making knowledgeable purchasers of health products and health services.

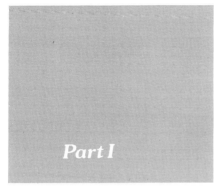

CONSUMER BEWARE!

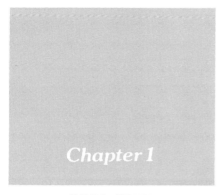

Chapter 1

QUACKERY

QUACKERY is the practicing of medicine, dentistry, or other accredited health profession by a dishonest or an incompetent person with little or no professional preparation to do what he claims he can do. The quack has a cure or treatment for every human disease, disability, or defect—and for a price.

Today's quack may be a house-to-house "doctor" who will, if permitted, invade the privacy of a home. He or she will discuss anyone's health needs. The quack will give advice and will sell a product.

The quack may run a special "clinic" outfitted with all the medical equipment found in the licensed medical doctor's examining room. It is not uncommon to find false diplomas. The quack may use the title, "doctor," and may wear a white jacket. He usually offers a "secret" formula to each customer, advertises special "cures," and provides the customer with a variety of services such as free lectures, books, or pamphlets, a variety of health foods, and quick cures. His products and services are advertised by radio, television, the press, and exhibits. If a quack is forced to stop his business, he moves to another state and starts again.

One of the biggest types of mail fraud is the mail-order practice operated by quacks. Some of the frauds are analysis of urine, diagnosis of cancer, devices to change the size and shape of the female breast, aids for sexual impotency, devices to treat arthritis, and cures for epilepsy. In one of the urinalysis-by-mail swindles, the customer was informed of his illnesses, even though the specimen of urine was not the customer's.

Fraud, theft, and death are the results of quackery. The customer who pays a large sum of money for a worthless product or "cure" is the victim of a *fraud*. At least 2 percent of our national budget goes into the pockets of quacks—outright *theft*. When the customer places his life in the hands of a quack who promises a cure, *death* may be the penalty the customer pays. Quacks deprive their customers of necessary medical care.

WHY QUACKERY EXISTS

Quackery exists for numerous reasons. Many people do not know the difference between a quack and a licensed medical doctor. Other persons would rather accept half-truths and misconceptions given by quacks than the truth from a medical doctor, particularly if they have a health disability with no known cure. Desperate persons such as parents with a child who has cancer will seek any means to prolong life.

Persons who have persistent anxieties about their health may be victims of quackery. These hypochondriacs believe they have illnesses or health conditions which medical doctors have assured them they do not have. The quack preys upon the hypochondriacs' anxieties and takes money for treating nonexistent illnesses or chronic health conditions.

A quack is always available when a medical doctor has given his patient no promise, no hope, no cure, and the truth about the patient's condition. The quack has some "cure," gives sympathy, listens to the customer, and assures the customer that the medical doctor was wrong. The quack has a product to sell at a special price, has testimonials claiming cures, and assures the customer that the product is sold under the quack's name.

A medical doctor may use laboratory tests and other medical diagnostic techniques before informing his patient of the diagnosis. A medical doctor sells no product under his name, has no shopper's special price, and has no testimonials. He will permit new medical information to be shared and evaluated by the American Medical Association, Federal Food and Drug Administration, National Institutes of Health, and pharmaceutical companies, along with societies of the medical specialists.

The most plausible reason for the existence of quackery is the consumer's lack of valid information about diseases, chronic health conditions, defects of some part of the human body, mental illness, obesity, disabilities from accidents, and general illnesses. The consumer asks: What is arthritis? Why, in this day of medical and technological advances, is there no treatment for arthritis? Why, in this day of "miracle" drugs, is there no medication to eradicate the pain accompanying arthritis? The consumer reads and hears about transplants of human organs and tissues, mechanical devices replacing the functions of an organ within the human body, and the testing of medications to insure effectiveness and safety. Thus, lacking valid health information and awed by the discoveries in health care, the consumer is an easy target for the quack.

ARTHRITIS

The number one crippler in the United States is arthritis which affects at least 13 million Americans. Most of these victims of arthritis are wracked with pain, and some are so disabled that they are unable to work, keep house, obtain an education, or engage in most recreational activities.

What Is Arthritis?

Arthritis is an inflammation of the joints with stiffness and aching in muscles, tendons, ligaments, and joints. The most common types of arthritis are osteoarthritis and rheumatoid arthritis.

Osteoarthritis. A health condition of overweight and elderly persons, osteoarthritis results from wear and tear on joints. The cartilage of the joints becomes damaged and disintegrates. Joints of the body show signs of wearing out because of the weight and use placed on them. Knees, ankles, hips, and vertebrae are changed by osteoarthritis due to pain, stiffness, and appearance of enlarged knobby joints.

Rheumatoid Arthritis. The majority of victims of rheumatoid arthritis are young and middle-aged adults. Children, too, are afflicted. Creeping up slowly on its victims, rheumatoid arthritis can cripple by attacking the joints and tissues around the joints. It can also damage organs such as the heart. Among the first signs of rheumatoid arthritis may be muscular stiffness, especially in the morning hours. Fatigue, loss of weight, and loss of appetite may appear.

Rheumatoid arthritis has a period of remission when the signs of the arthritis disappear. This remission period follows a period of time when there was severe fever and badly inflamed joints. During the remission, the victim feels well.

The medical care of the arthritic victim consists of prescribed medication, rest, and exercise under the supervision of a physician. The main aim of the medical care is the prevention of joint destruction. Physical therapy is administered for the maintenance of joint function and for strengthening the muscles that support the joints. Prescribed medication usually reduces the inflammation at the joints. Rest is particularly important when the joints are inflamed and painful. Research continuously probes for ways to control arthritis.

Arthritis Quackery

Because there is no known cure for arthritis and there is a period of remission, quacks thrive on arthritis victims. The intense pain accompanying arthritis makes the victims easy prey for the arthritis quack and his "cures."

Most painkillers recommended by quacks are over-the-counter drugs having aspirin and caffeine as their chief ingredients. Aspirin may supress pain and inflammation, but there is no evidence that caffeine enhances the effect of aspirin. Most painkillers are only temporary measures and seldom reduce the swelling and inflammation at the joints.

Some of the nostrums for the cure of arthritis offered by quacks are sea salts, uranium ore, bee venom, and olive oil. One nostrum advocated in the 1960's was repeated injections of bee venom. The use of bee venom for painful joints stems from an old European folk belief rejected by medical authorities as a treatment of arthritis. Another arthritis quack prescribed drinking cod-liver oil with orange juice and a dietary regimen that avoided water at meals. Among the nostrums for arthritis has been moon dust supposedly brought to earth by astronauts. Rubbing the dust on a joint would cure arthritis. Uranium ore has been sold in mitts or pads filled with low-grade ore, or the arthritis victim has paid an exorbitant price to sit in a pit of uranium ore that purportedly emitted "healing radiations." One pad seized by the Food and Drug Administration emitted less radioactivity than a luminous watch dial.

Some of the gadgets sold by quacks are copper bracelets, cloth mittens with electrical wiring, harnesses to stretch the limbs, and vibrators. Copper bracelets are worn around the wrists, arms, ankles, and legs to prevent swelling of joints. Sellers of cloth mittens with electrical wiring have guaranteed that the wearer would have less arthritic pain. Promoters of harnesses to stretch the neck, spinal vertebrae, legs, and arms have promised the arthritic victim that the swelling at the joints would be reduced. Vibrators such as a vibrating mattress have proven to be dangerous to victims of rheumatoid arthritis. Many expensive mechanical gadgets that have been promoted as cures for arthritis have been seized by the Food and Drug Administration.

"Secret formulas" have been sold as medications. Often the secret formulas would be dangerous hormones and drugs seldom used by medical doctors. Promoters of "immune milk" from cows injected with "vaccines" containing streptococci and staphylococci claimed that these cows produced antibodies which would immunize rheumatoid arthritis victims. The price for "immune milk" ranged from one to two dollars a quart. Recently "immune milk" has again appeared as a special dietary supplement. Another secret formula was a home-brewed hormone, which, according to the promoter, could wipe out the pain and swelling of arthritis.

Special baths, including sauna baths, are also promoted as cures for arthritis. Sauna baths introduce intense heat to the human body so that normal body temperature rises and produces excessive perspiration. The arthritic victim taking a sauna bath loses a considerable amount of water and mineral salts through perspiration. The proprietors of spas and mineral baths advertise cures for arthritis on the theory that arthritis is caused by constipation or toxemia. Arthritis caused by constipation or toxemia has been disproven by medical authorities.

"Miracle cures" of the quack have been given in testimonials of arthritis victims. Because of the periods of remission, the "miracle cure" completely restored the arthritis victim to good health. These cures have been proven worthless by the Federal Food and Drug Administration and the Arthritis Foundation. A community voluntary health agency, the Foundation has indicated that it is no longer a question of whether arthritis will be controlled, but *when* it will be controlled.

CANCER

Knowledge of the need for early detection of cancer has resulted in more than 1.5 million living American successfully "cured" of cancer. Cancer strikes at any age. One in four Americans will have cancer. Some victims will seek cancer quacks because of fear and ignorance of cancer.

Cancers of the Human Body

Normal cells are similar in physical structure and in functions. These cells divide in an orderly manner into specific tissues and organs with designated functions. Normal cell growth ceases when its purpose has been achieved.

Abnormal cells are not fully understood. These cells grow and reproduce in a disorderly, uncontrolled manner. One cell may become three, eight, or more cells, and be irregular in size and shape. These abnormal cells do not assume the functions of normal cells and may grow in many parts of the body.

When abnormal cells confine themselves to a limited area and do not spread to other parts of the human body, these abnormal cells are a benign cell growth. When abnormal cells spread to surrounding tissues and continue to multiply, these abnormal cells are a malignant cell growth. This is cancer. If not checked, the abnormal cells can penetrate the blood stream and the lymph channels which will carry them to other parts of the human body where they establish colonies. Control of cancer thus depends upon early detection before the abnormal cells are disseminated throughout the body.

At least 200 to 300 kinds of cancer occur in man, with 30 common types accounting for 90 percent of the human cancers. Human cancers may be found in the skin, mouth, nose and sinuses, pharynx, larynx, lung, stomach, colon, rectum, breast, uterus, bladder, prostate, bone, blood, and lymph. Cancers have been found also in human eyeballs, the brain, penis and testicles, and kidneys.

Each of these human cancers has distinct warning signals. Among the warning signals of possible uterine cancer are unusual bleeding and discharges from the vagina. Warning signals of possible prostate cancer are a weak or interrupted flow of urine, inability to urinate or to start urinating, need to urinate frequently at night, blood in the urine, and difficulty in stopping the flow of urine.

Recognition of the warning signals of cancer makes early detection possible. Any of the following conditions should be called to the attention of a physician.

1. Unusual bleeding or discharges.
2. A lump or thickening in the breast or elsewhere.
3. A sore that does not heal.
4. Change in bowel or bladder habits.
5. Hoarseness or cough.
6. Indigestion or difficulty in swallowing.
7. Change in size or color of a wart or mole.

An annual medical examination, an annual dental examination, breast self-examination by women, the "Pap" test, blood tests, specimens of body tissues and urine, and chest roentgenograms of the lungs of smokers can assist the physician in detecting early cancers of the human body.

Early detection of cancers has saved many patients' lives. Physicians can successfully treat cancers by surgery, radiation, and chemotherapy. Research is continuously finding new methods for the treatment of cancer.

Cancer Quackery

"Cancer clinics," various concoctions, special vaccines, anticancer drugs, diets, mechanical gadgets, and other worthless cures are some of the types of cancer quackery available to the gullible customer. The so-called cancer clinics, such as the Hoxsey Cancer Clinic of Dallas, Texas, were well-advertised. The Hoxsey method of treating cancer consisted of internal medicine taken orally as a liquid or a pill and containing potassium iodide combined with red clover, prickly ash bark, licorice, and different roots and barks. In addition, a yellow powder, a red paste, or a clear solution, depending upon the type and location of the cancer, was prescribed for external application. The supportive treatment prescribed was a combination of vitamins, iron supplements, antacids, diuretics, and laxatives. Although routine urine and blood examinations were made along with roentgenograms of each patient, no licensed medical doctor was associated with the "clinic." For at least ten years, the Food and Drug Administration pursued its case to close the Hoxsey Cancer Clinics, not only in Dallas but also in other cities. To reach the public, the Food and Drug Administration posted a warning in post offices and postal substations that the Hoxsey methods for treating cancer were worthless and dangerous.[1,2]

Red clover, alfalfa, fig juice, prickly ash bark, and honey drip cane, either as powders or liquids, are some of the concoctions that have been prescribed by cancer quacks as internal remedies for cancer. Bamfolin, an extract from the leaf of one species of bamboo grass, was another so-called cure. The grass was crushed, cooked with calcium lye, and extracted with alcohol. A powder of pure diamonds constituted the formula of the Diamond Carbon Compound claimed to cure cancer. For cancer on the skin, the Compound was mixed with lime water.[3] Often the concoctions consisted of water, vinegar, molasses, or baking soda and water in addition to the "secret formula." One quack charged $500 for his cancer "cure." When the "cure" was analyzed by the Food and Drug Administration, it was found to be water straight from the faucet.

The Frost method used special vaccines and diet. The vaccines were made of the patient's own fluids, Staphylococci aureus, and certain antibiotics. Staphylococcus aureus is the causative agent of various staphylococci diseases and is found in skin lesions such as boils, abscesses, infected lacerations, impetigo, and carbuncles. It is often the cause of staphylococcal diseases in hospital nurseries. The American Cancer Society found no evidence that these vaccines were effective treatments for cancer.[4] Until the specific causative agent of a particular type of cancer can be found, no vaccine for that type of cancer can be available.

Many anticancer drugs have been proposed for the treatment of cancer. Some of these have been Anticancergen Z-50, a biological preparation which was administered intramuscularly. Antineol was a preparation described to be extracted from the posterior lobe of the pituitary gland of cattle. Laetrile was an empirical drug derived from apricot kernels. The promoter of Laetrile claimed it released cyanide to cancers of the human body. Iscador was a preparation made from various kinds of mistletoe. Polonine, as described by its discoverer, was a combination of organic acids and antiseptics reacting with vitamins to produce salts.[5] All of these anticancer drugs were proven worthless.

Possibly the best publicized anticancer drug was krebiozen. Considered as "one of the greatest frauds of the 20th century," krebiozen was produced originally by Stevan Durovic, M.D., a Yugoslavian physician. The original formula was an extract of the blood of 2,000 Argentine horses injected with the microorganism causing "lumpy jaw" in cattle. This formula was brought to the United States at which time Dr. Durovic was joined by Dr. Andrew C. Ivy, a prestigious medical scientist and vice president of one of the largest universities of higher learning. After gathering data of the effects by krebiozen as an anticancer drug taken by 22 patients, Dr. Ivy committed his reputation to the promotion of krebiozen, against the advice of other medical scientists. When the Food and Drug Administration tested its effectiveness as an anticancer drug, krebiozen was found to be creatine, an amino acid derivative found in meat of the ordinary diet, and a normal body component. Krebiozen has not proven to be effective in the treatment of cancers of the human body.[6]

Diets advocated by quacks to cure cancer may exclude meat, eggs, fruits, milk, vegetables, or cereals. The Grape Diet, for example, has been used to treat cancer by naturopaths, promoters of health spas, and cancer quacks. Starting at 8:00 A.M. and repeated every two hours, the cancer victim was instructed to eat fresh grapes weighing from two ounces to half a pound. Only water was added to the diet. Unsweetened grape juice could be substituted for grapes, or if the fresh grapes were not available, unsulfured raisins were added to the grape juice. All grape products were sold in health food stores. External cancers were treated with grape poultices. Grape juice gargles and enemas or douches were also used, depending upon the types of human cancers.[7] Any one food or a special diet of certain foods may be promoted as a cure for cancers by quacks.

Many types of mechanical gadgets with electrical switches and colored lights, indicators, knobs, and scientific sounding names have been advertised to cure cancers. With some of the gadgets were metal plates to be attached to the part of the human body afflicted by cancer. These plates were to carry vibrations to cure the cancer. Other gadgets had belts that held the customer close to the miracle-curing machinery. Some quacks sold gadgets that could be plugged into an electrical outlet for home self-cures for cancers.

Although not outrightly claiming to cure cancer, commercialized faith healers have advertised prayer cloths which, when worn next to the human body, will cure any disease. The commercialized faith healer tells the victim of cancer that he (the healer) has prayed over the cloth, which, if purchased, will heal.

Worthless tonics may not be advertised as cures for cancer, but claims made for them may lead the gullible customer to believe that the tonic can cure or prevent cancer. Claims that the tonic will provide "good health" and "rid the body of suffering" may be promoted in an extravaganza of newspaper and television advertising. One such product, Hadacol, had cash sales during one year of 75 million dollars. Hadacol, which was promoted by a Louisiana state senator, Dudley J. LeBlanc, sold for $1.25 for an 8-ounce bottle or $3.50 for the 24-ounce, "family economy size." It consisted of a mixture of some B complex vitamins, iron, calcium, phosphorus, honey, dilute hydrochloric acid, and 12 percent alcohol. The American Medical Association's Council on Pharmacy and Chemistry and its Bureau of Investigation released information to its member physicians that Hadacol was not a specific medication and was not a specific preventive measure.[8] Other tonics that have been advertised to promote "good health" infer that the customer will have a long life, free of cancer.

The American Cancer Society has compiled numerous unproven methods for cancer treatment. Among those have been Pangametin, Cancer Lipid Concentrate, Carcin, Carzodelan, Coley's Mixed Toxins, Fresh Cell Therapy, The Gerson Method, Gibson Methods, the Glover Serum, Koch Antitoxins, Mucorhicin, Revici Cancer Control, Spears Hygienic System, and Staphylococcus Phage Lysates.[9]

COSMETIC QUACKERY

Since the beginning of time, men and women have desired concoctions to remove wrinkles from the face, restore hair to bald scalps, rebuild sagging features of the jaws, and appear younger. Whether the woman was Bathsheba or the daughter of Herodias, the lotions used to enhance her beauty were carefully guarded secrets. The beauty of Helen of Troy was told in songs and legends of the early Greeks. As the Romans conquered foreign lands, they sought the strange potions and poultices claimed to restore beauty and youth. Cleopatra's beauty so entranced Julius Caesar and Marc Anthony that the Roman empire felt its impact. Not only women but also men searched for ways to appear younger and to be more attractive. Henry VIII and the male aristocrats of France and Italy prized their wigs and facial creams as much as their art treasures. Explorers to the New World sought mystical waters to restore the middle-aged man to his youth. Today, cosmetic quacks enjoy lucrative profits because of each person's desire to look younger and to be beautiful or handsome.

Skin

No cosmetic product will cure skin disorders or restore youthfulness to aging skin. Beauty cannot be bought. Every consumer should be skeptical of elaborate claims made by advertisers of beauty products. With a little knowledge of the structure of the skin, the consumer will be better able to evaluate the advertising claims made for cosmetics.

The skin has three layers. The epidermis is the tough outer layer consisting of dead and new cells. The dead cells are constantly being shed and replaced by new cells. The second layer is the true skin or dermis which is composed of blood vessels, sense organs, small bundles of smooth muscles, sweat and oil glands, hair follicles, and fat cells. There are two sets of sweat glands found all over the body. The eccrine glands secrete sweat which cools the body by evaporation. The apocrine glands, found near hair follicles, have a chemical affinity to certain sex hormones. The oil glands secrete sebum which helps to keep the skin and hair soft, waterproof, and pliable. Also within the dermis is a network of elastic and nonelastic fibers which lose their elasticity with age. Thus, creases are formed by folds in the skin which remain instead of being ironed out smoothly. These creases are wrinkles. The third layer is the subcutaneous layer composed of fat and elastic fibers. This layer is a storage place for fat, a heat regulator, and a protector for nerves and blood vessels. The contour of the body is determined by this layer.

The shelves of any drugstore are crowded with products for skin care. There are analgesic liquids, poultices, ointments, and balms; acne remedies; medicated bath preparations, creams, lotions, and powders; antipruritics (itch remedies); skin healing preparations; eczema remedies; germicidal soaps; hormone creams; psoriasis remedies; seborrhea balms; wart removers; fungicides; lip pomades; facial balms; blemish removers;

sunburn remedies; and cleansers and other preparations for customers to spray, rub, or pour on their skins.

A variety of suntan products are bought by the consumer—creams, oils, jellies, lotions, aerosol foams, and ointments. Some of the less desirable products are suntan pills containing chemicals to prevent and reduce sunburn. Most dermatologists indicate that the chemicals found in these suntan pills are dangerous for self-use.

Chemical tanners may leave an artificial stain. The chemical, dihydroxyacetone, has been used in most tanning products. This chemical may cause the skin to have a yellowish tinge, irritate acne, produce an allergic reaction, and wear off within a few days. Too often, many persons cannot accept that they do not tan or that tanning takes gradual sun exposures over a period of time. No suntan product can produce a tan of the skin if the skin will not tan. Tanning the skin is not done in one day.

Hormone creams have been promoted by manufacturers of cosmetic products. Research has established that estrogen, when rubbed on the skin of *some* women, has produced a *small* increase in the cells of the dermis and a *slight* increase in the blood supply to the skin. Utilizing these facts, the manufacturers of cosmetic products have advertised that the hormone creams can keep the complexion beautiful and the face youthful. Other hormone creams have contained pregnenolone acetate which when tested by the Food and Drug Administration revealed unexpected hazards. Many of the hormone creams are unsafe for some women.

Cosmetic manufacturers have advertised royal jelly as a cure-all for skin disorders and aging. A substance supplied from the glands of worker bees and fed to the female larvae, royal jelly has long been touted for its restorative powers for human beings (Fig. 1-1). Royal jelly is available as lotions, injections, soaps, and capsules, but it has no therapeutic value.

Turtle oil, buttermilk, shark oil, extract of placenta, and rose petals have been advertised to remove wrinkles, retard aging, and restore a beautiful complexion. None of the advertising claims made for these products or combinations of these products have been proven.

Deodorants and antiperspirants have astronomical sales, since advertisers have made the American public "body-odor conscious." Body odor is caused by the action of bacteria on secretions from the eccrine sweat glands, apocrine sweat glands, and sebaceous glands. The secretions from these glands, except possibly those of the apocrine glands, are odorless before they are exposed to the skin and the air. Scientists have concluded that substances within the ducts of the glands, have decomposed and are spread over the skin surface. To get rid of body odor, either bacterial action must be stopped or secretions from these glands must be reduced. Deodorant soaps and deodorants may reduce the bacterial

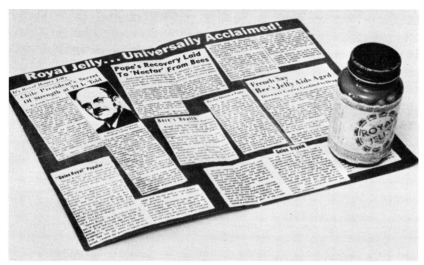

FIGURE 1-1

Examples of news stories about royal jelly. (Courtesy of the Food and Drug Administration, Dallas, Texas.)

action. Antiperspirants may reduce both bacterial action and secretions from sweat glands. The labels for antiperspirants and deodorants must show their active ingredients, since these drugs are under the Federal Food, Drug, and Cosmetic Act. The labels for deodorants should make no claim about controlling perspiration. The best way to control bacterial growth on the skin and body odor is regular bathing with a thorough cleansing of all parts of the skin. For longer-lasting protection against bacteria in the underarm area, a daily bath with thorough skin cleaning and a deodorant containing an antiseptic sprayed on the underarm area may be the best protection.

Self-medication for acne is not uncommon among high school youth, since cosmetic quacks advertise a variety of useless vaccines, vitamins, tablets, pills, cleaning pastes, and foam aerosols as cures for acne. Often the high school youth has little understanding of acne. Sebaceous glands secrete sebum, a fatty and waxlike material, into the upper portion of the hair follicles which form skin pores. When these pores become clogged, the sebum cannot escape to the skin surface, and the lesions of acne appear. Acne is an unsightly skin condition with blemishes, blackheads, and pimples. Some simple rules in preventing severe cases of acne are:

1. Pimples and blackheads should not be squeezed.
2. Skin areas affected with acne should be washed with thick soapsuds three or four times a day.
3. Warm towels should be applied to the affected skin area after washing.

Many teenage girls and women use face creams instead of soap and water for cleansing the face. These creams may plug the skin pores and aggravate the acne. A physician can prescribe drugs and proprietary remedies and indicate the care of the skin to meet the specific needs of the person with acne.

Another skin disorder for which cosmetic quacks offer a wide variety of products is eczema. A red, scaly, swollen area that tends to have a clear fluid is probably eczema. This fluid dries into scales or crusts which may or may not itch. Self-medication with some cure-all can aggravate the condition. Often the user of the cure-all does not understand that the skin will heal if the inflamed area is kept dry and he avoids substances that irritate the skin.

Recently advertisers have promoted vitamin E for scars, dry skin, facial lines, wrinkles, and aging skin. The skin lotions and creams are advertised as producing "incredible" and "amazing" results. To date, vitamin E as a therapeutic cosmetic has not been reported in the *Archives of Dermatology, Journal of Investigative Dermatology,* or *British Journal of Dermatology.* Also, vitamin E has been publicized as a deodorant. The theory is that vitamin E stops bacteria from utilizing oxygen to break down secretions of underarm pores which become odorous.

Hair and Scalp

All types of expensive treatments, appliances, and gadgets have been placed against the scalp to induce hair to grow. Cosmetic quacks have methods to remove unwanted hair on the underarms and legs. Advertised dandruff "cures" have made the American public acutely aware of dandruff. The consumer who knows about the structure of the hair and scalp is better able to evaluate hair and scalp products.

Hair follicles, embedded in the dermis and extending to the outer edge of the epidermis, hold hairs. Cells at the base of these follicles supply new hairs when old hairs are cut away or drop out. The shaft is the part of the hair above the skin surface. The root is below the skin surface. The hair consists of compacted layers and resembles the outer layer of the skin in structure. The pigment in one of the layers gives the hair its color. Baldness is believed to be due to some hereditary factor or possibly to sex hormones.

Hair restorers, expensive treatments, massage gadgets, and cure-alls will not cause hair to grow on the scalp. Baldness cannot be cured by remedies of quacks. If a man wants to hide his baldness, he can wear a wig or toupee.

Gray hair is due to the reduction of pigment in the hair. The hair colorants widely used by both sexes can affect the hair's structure to some extent, can cause some damage to the hair when the colorants are continuously used, may bring about a skin reaction, and often do not hide the gray hair appearing at the roots. All types of terms are placed on the labels of hair colorants: tints, rinses, dyes, temporary and permanent colorants, and bleaches. Before any hair colorant is used, a small amount of the colorant, in the same concentration as when applied to the hair, should be placed on some part of the skin and left undisturbed for 24 hours. After that period the skin under the colorant should show no sign of irritation. If a hair colorant is used, a touch-up is needed regularly at the roots and a complete re-dyeing several times a year. Cosmetic quacks offer products claimed to keep the hair the same color for many years without any touch-up and re-dyeing.

Too much hair in the area of the underarms and on the legs can be unsightly for women. Shaving, depilatories, and electrolysis are methods for removing such hair. Both shaving and depilatories remove the shafts of unwanted hair without affecting the hair growth. Some chemical depilatories may cause injury to the skin if the depilatory is left on the skin for longer than the specified time. Others use chemicals creating skin reactions. If the follicle from which the hair grows is to be completely destroyed, electrolysis is the answer, but it should be done by a dermatologist. During electrolysis, superfluous hair can be permanently removed, leaving no scar or trace of any unwanted hair. Electric devices sold by quacks for home treatment to remove excess hair should be avoided.

The scalp, like the skin of other parts of the body, continuously sloughs off bits of its dead outer layer. Some oiliness and flakiness of the scalp are normal. Extra sebaceous glands in the scalp may produce an excessive amount of oily secretion. Combined with dirt in the air and excessive sweating, this oily secretion forms large flakes that hang loosely in the hair. Excessive scaling of the scalp is dandruff, which may be accompanied by itching.

Even though no complete method for the prevention of dandruff is available, all types of products are offered to prevent and cure dandruff. Shampooing the hair more frequently than once a week, even daily, will reduce the dandruff and not harm the scalp or hair. Severe dandruff should be called to the attention of a dermatologist. One misconception about dandruff is that it causes male baldness.

Eyes

Studies by ophthalmologists and the Food and Drug Administration have revealed that eye cosmetics need to be handled with extreme care. A mascara brush can scratch the cornea and infect the cornea with a type of bacteria that can cause eye infections. These bacteria, *Pseudomonas*, and other microorganisms can lead to serious inflammation of the surface of the eyeball and blindness. The human eyeball is bathed by its own secretions which keep in balance the microorganisms which reach the underside of the eyelid and the surface of the eyeball. When additional microorganisms are introduced by use of contaminated eye cosmetics, the possibility of infection is greatly increased. Even though the cosmetic manufacturer may include a preservative to retard the growth of the microorganisms, the eye cosmetic may be misused by the consumer. In addition to eye cosmetics are ophthalmic preparations sold as over-the-counter drugs. In one FDA study of eye ointments, microbial contamination was evident. According to FDA regulations both ophthalmic drugs and cosmetic-type liquid eye products to refresh tired eyes must be sterile. However, the eye drugs must be properly used and kept free from contamination by the consumer. In the use of eye cosmetics, the FDA offers the following suggestions.

1. Discontinue use of any eye product if that product causes irritation, and see a physician.
2. Wash hands before applying the eye cosmetic, since the hands contain microorganisms.
3. Be sure that any instrument placed in the eye or around the eyeball is clean.
4. Do not allow eye cosmetics to become covered with dust or contaminated with dirt.
5. Do not use old containers for eye cosmetics.
6. Do not spit into eye cosmetics. Use boiled water to moisten eye cosmetic.
7. Do not share your eye cosmetics.
8. Do not store eye cosmetics at temperatures above 85° F because of deterioration of the preservative.
9. Avoid using eye cosmetics if there is an eye infection or an inflammation of the skin around the eye.
10. Take care in the use of eye cosmetics if you have any allergies.
11. Be careful not to scratch the eyeball when removing eye cosmetics.[10]

Cosmetic quacks may promote eye washes, along with other cosmetics to "refresh" the eyes. No synthetic product can match the natural fluids of the eyeball. These fluids not only wash away small particles of dust and other irritating materials but also contain mild bacteria-destroying properties beneficial to the eyeball. However, the consumer of the quack eye washes uses these products when there are indications of infections, itching, and burning sensation of the eyeball and eyelids, rather than seeking the medical care of a physician. Many of these consumers of the quack eye products may have glaucoma—intense intraocular pressure of the eyeball and cupping of the optic disc. Pain in and around the eyeball, loss of side vision, eye aches after seeing movies or television in the dark, and fuzzy or blurred vision are some of the signs of glaucoma. Many victims of glaucoma that resulted in blindness were unaware of the dangers of glaucoma and the need for medical care. In addition, eye fatigue not associated with glaucoma may result from farsightedness, nearsightedness, or astigmatism. No quack eye wash can retard the damage to the eyeball by glaucoma or correct errors in eye refraction.

DENTAL QUACKERY

Exaggerated advertising claims based on inadequate research are made for many dentifrices, mouth washes, cheap flase teeth, "treatments" for poorly fitting teeth and gum diseases, devices to fluoridate home water supplies, fluoride supplements, and other dental preparations and gadgets. The buyers include the more than 100,000 American teenagers who are completely edentulous (toothless); other teenagers who have 14 decayed, missing, or filled teeth; the 20-year-old college student with periodontal diseases; and the 30-year-old successful executive with complete dentures. As with products for the care of the skin and the hair, the consumer who has some knowledge of the causes and treatment of tooth decay, periodontal diseases, and malocclusion and of regulatory agencies is better able to recognize the dental quack.

Dental caries is a destructive and progressive process that produces cavities in the teeth and destroys tooth structure. Four factors contribute to produce dental caries: (1) presence of decay-producing bacteria, (2) diet with large amounts of sugar, (3) dental plaque, and (4) a susceptible tooth surface. The bacteria multiply into bacterial colonies called plaque. Colorless and transparent, the plaque is constantly sticking to the teeth. When the bacteria come in contact with foods with large amounts of sugar, more plaque is produced and the bacteria act on the sugar to produce acids. These acids begin to dissolve the enamel of the tooth and start decay. Even without plaque, caries can develop, since food residues collect in pits and fissures of the teeth. Left undetected, the decay will penetrate the enamel, reach the dentin, and invade the pulp cavity. When the pulp cavity becomes infected, an abscess may form resulting in the loss of the tooth and/or caries in adjoining teeth.

Loss of teeth may be due to periodontal diseases. Gums become tender, inflamed, and swollen in gingivitis. The gums bleed easily and stand away from the teeth. Deposits of plaque and other mouth conditions cause gingivitis. When gingivitis is neglected, periodontitis (pyorrhea) results. Gums separate from the teeth, leaving pockets into which food particles can accumulate. These food particles decay in the pockets and pus forms. As periodontitis becomes worse, the pockets deepen, more pus forms, gums bleed, and tissue damage increases. In the final stages, the bone which supports the tooth is attacked and destroyed. The result is a loose permanent tooth which comes out.

Often the adult not only has caries and periodontal disease but also has malocclusion. Malocclusion is an abnormal occlusal relationship because of irregularities in the positions and contacts of the teeth when the jaws are closed. It may occur during the time the deciduous teeth are being shed and the permanent teeth are erupting.

Professional dental care during the shedding of the deciduous teeth and the eruption of the permanent teeth would correct malocclusion. Continuous professional dental care throughout a lifetime would insure reduction of loss of teeth from dental caries and periodontal diseases. Proper tooth brushing, use of dental disclosing materials, diets low in sugar content, fluoridation of community water supplies, and avoidance of dental quacks with their products would reduce the number of customers of dental quackery.

The dental quack may advertise locally or contact his customers on a house-to-house basis. Some dental quacks maintain a poorly equipped laboratory or dental office with false diplomas hanging on the walls. The proprietors of such unethical establishments usually advertise their services and products and label their offices as laboratories. The American Dental Association has identified these quacks as bootleg dentists or bushwackers.

The Council on Dental Therapeutics, American Dental Association, evaluates most dental health products available to the American consumer. Among these products are dentifrices—toothpastes and tooth powders. The Council requires all dentifrices to undergo thorough and lengthy clinical testing to substantiate the claims of the dentifrice manufacturer, particularly if those claims include therapeutic or prophylactic effects. After the clinical testing, the dentifrice is placed in one of four classifications:

A Accepted.

B Provisionally accepted.

C The evidence is so limited and so inconclusive that the product cannot be accurately evaluated.

D Unacceptable because of inability to meet the standards in the provision for acceptance.

If therapeutic claims are made on the label of a dentifrice, the Federal Food and Drug Administration has made additional tests to insure the dentifrice's safety and effectiveness. The Food and Drug Administration can remove the dentifrice from sale if the label has therapeutic claims which have not been proven by the FDA's tests.

Dentrifices are among the products advertised by the illicit dentist. The consumer should be wary when any of the following claims are made:

1. Dentifrices that remineralize the teeth.

2. Dentifrices that remove or retard calculus (layer of living bacterial plaque on the crown surfaces of the teeth or the root surfaces beneath the gum margins. Calculus has rough, rocklike edges making it easier for plaque to accumulate.)

3. Dentifrices with foaming agents for "antibacterial" activity.

4. Dentifrices with chlorophyll.

5. Dentifrices containing urea and types of ammonia phosphates.

6. Dentifrices with hexachlorophene.

The dental quack may have a mouthwash to "remove all bacteria from the mouth" or "prevent tooth decay." Most mouthwashes with therapeutic claims have been evaluated by the Council on Dental Therapeutics, American Dental Association and have been classified as D— Unacceptable. Mouth odor or bad breath may be due to lack of proper tooth brushing or no tooth brushing, lack of professional dental care, too many foods high in sugar content, use of tobacco and/or alcoholic beverages, indigestion, diseases of the nose and mouth, focal infections in the throat or some part of the digestive system, periodontal diseases, or other infections causing expectorations from the mouth. Proper tooth brushing before retiring will reduce the amount of mouth bacteria and food particles on the teeth. Plain water used as a rinse can wash away food particles. The mouthwash with the smell of mint or other nonoffensive aroma hides the bad breath for only a short period of time.

Cheap artificial teeth are often provided by quacks to gullible customers. Often called "store-bought," these teeth permit the customer to fit certain sizes of dentures to his mouth. When the customer finds a denture that fits snugly, he believes he has a set of teeth which will allow him to bite, chew, and tear food. After the purchase, the customer finds that the store-bought teeth cannot be used to bite, chew, and tear food.

Often accompanying the cheap artificial teeth are adhesive preparations to hold the dentures tightly against the gums. Many of these adhesive preparations are health hazards because they contain substances that irritate the gums. Some persons may suffer dermatitis, eczema, or gastrointestinal distress from the ingredients in adhesive preparations.[11] Many have no therapeutic values for the gum tissues. The preparations may actually be harmful because they create a false sense of retention and encourage the customer to wear the denture for long periods with no check of the fit of the denture base to the gums.

Treatments for gum diseases may be provided by the dental quack. Often they consist of applications of antibiotics or salt solutions without regard for the type of periodontal disease or other diseases of the mouth or throat. In some instances the treatment has been directions mailed to the customer.

Devices to fluoridate home water supplies have been promoted by dental quacks. These devices sold at exorbitant prices have been proven useless because the amount of fluorine varies in different local water supplies. If the community has controlled fluoridation of water supplies, one part of fluorine is added to one million parts of water. If the community has uncontrolled fluoridation or natural fluoridation of water supplies, the amount of fluorine may exceed one part of fluorine to one million parts of water. It is possible that the community may have less than one part of fluorine to one million parts of water.

The Council on Dental Therapeutics, American Dental Association, has not accepted fluoride supplements. The indiscriminate use of dietary sodium fluoride by individuals living in communities with varying amount of fluoride in the community water supplies has made the dosage of the fluoride supplement highly questionable. Dietary fluoride supplement requires careful supervision to maintain consistent and continuous administration and to avoid mottling of the enamel, or dental fluorosis. Dietary sodium fluoride advocated by the dental quack should be avoided. Topical fluoride applications by the family dentist to teeth of children in early childhood, however, may reduce caries 30 to 40 percent.

Some dental quacks sell devices and gadgets ranging from electric toothbrushes to water irrigators. Regardless of the status of the person's dental health, the device or gadget is promoted as a cure for the dental problem. The customer may accept the false claims because of a money-back guarantee. Only the so-called dentist profits.

MECHANICAL QUACKERY

All types of electrical machinery, devices, and gadgets have been sold by quacks to cure diseases, chronic health conditions, injuries, or mental illness. Outlandish prices are charged by mechanotherapists, naturopaths, and sanipractors for gadgets that usually can be made for a few dollars. Some quacks promote electronic diagnosis and treatment without any information about the customer. Others claim that vibrations come from expensive mechanical devices.

The founder of the fraudulent electrotherapy cult was Albert Abrams.[12] A medical doctor regarded by his colleagues as "money-mad," Abrams developed a "new" medical system which would correct malfunctioning of various organs and tissues of the human body by the excitation of certain centers of the spinal cord. He promoted the term, *spondylotherapy,* and held courses of spondylotherapy for which he charged $200. "Electronic Reactions of Abrams" was based on the theory that electrons, not the cell, form the real basis of life and that electrons are the sources of diseases. He devised a Dynamizer to diagnose the disease of a customer from a drop of blood sent to Abrams. His Ossillocast, a cure-all gadget containing electrical wires in a sealed box purportedly gave out vibrations to destroy diseases. It was leased for $1000 to $2000 a week. Another gadget, ERA, offered diagnosis and cure of any ailment. Later, the ERA was labeled "radionics." Abrams proposed he could determine the diseases of any person by that person's handwriting or blood sample. Customers were encouraged to send drops of blood on blotters, along with $10, to have their diseases or ailments diagnosed. At one time, ERA practioners numbered 3500 throughout many countries.

Physicians seeking to expose the mechanical quackery of Abrams found patients healthy whom Abrams' ERA methods had diagnosed as having syphilis. In one instance, a drop of blood on blotting paper was sent to Abrams who diagnosed the blood as coming from a patient having malaria, syphilis, diabetes, and cancer. The blood sample was from a young Plymouth Rock rooster.

It was estimated that Abrams grossed between two and five million dollars during the promotion of his mechanical quackery. As a result of his success, mechanotherapists and electrotherapists formed such companies as the Electronic Medical Foundation, International Electronic Research Foundation, and Drown Laboratories. The Electronic Medical Foundation marketed some 5000 of Abrams' mechanical devices. Twenty-eight varieties of Abrams-type gadgets emerged. One customer paid $28,600 for a worthless machine to cure a nervous ailment. Sanipractors, licensed drugless healers, used mechanical quackery of many varieties. Micro-Dynameters, used for diagnosing the customer's illness while the customer held two electrodes, were distributed to 5000 mechanical quacks.

The Food and Drug Administration has destroyed thousands of phony diagnostic and treatment devices used by mechanical quacks (Fig. 1-2). However, the Food and Drug Administration needs the assistance of

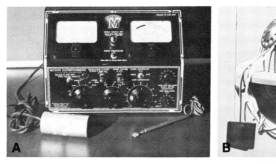
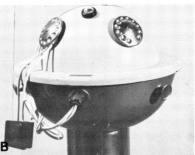
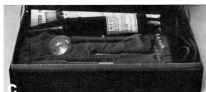
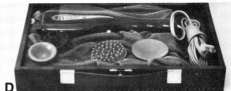

FIGURE 1-2

Examples of devices seized by the Food and Drug Administration. A. This device advertised for diagnosing and treating various disorders was merely a galvanometer that registers the amount of moisture in the skin. B. This device, which converted household current into a stimulation voltage, was advertised as effective for toning, strengthening, and rejuvenating the body, removing wrinkles, correcting fallen arches, and treating cancer. C. A violet ray device that was promoted as treatment to stimulate any muscle or nerve, especially the nerve centers at the base of the spine. D. A vibrator that was promoted for the treatment of colds, nervousness, throbbing headaches, tiredness, eye strain, insomnia, indigestion, constipation, and several other ailments and conditions. (Courtesy of the Food and Drug Administration, Dallas, Texas.)

state agencies charged with licensing health practioners using mechanical quackery. The Drown Laboratories has been an example of how the State of California took action against mechanical quackery.

The Drown Laboratories treated some 35,000 customers from whom they received a half million dollars. Devices used by the operators of the Drown Laboratories were claimed to diagnose and cure every known ailment from emotional illness to cancer and diseases and defects that medical science had not discovered. Many customers paid $588 for the Drown Therapeutic Instrument to treat themselves at home. For $35 a month the customer could send a blood specimen to the Drown Laboratories where the specimens were "analyzed" in one of the machines. In promotional material the Drown Laboratories offered to send an "hour's worth of treatment" to the customer anywhere on the face of the earth. Other machines using a process of "radio-vision" were claimed to be able to take photographs of diseased organs of customers by remote control, wherever the customer lived. Dr. Ruth Drown, the chief owner of Drown Laboratories, claimed that jazz music was a cause of cancer and that cancer could be prevented by listening to soothing music. Also, she expounded the theory that the human body was surrounded by a magnetic field. In her publication *Drown Atlas of Radio Therapy* she revealed that a person taking a shower bath would have his magnetic field washed down the drain.

An undercover agent for the California State Department of Public Health took three blood samples to the Drown Laboratories. The blood samples came from a sheep, a turkey, and a pig. The undercover agent paid $50 for the diagnosis of each blood sample and was told that the blood samples indicated that the "children" from whom the samples came would have mumps and chicken pox. In addition to the undercover agent's account of "diagnosis" from the Drown Laboratories, another witness for the state told the court that Dr. Drown claimed she could cure him of epilepsy.[13] The State of California arrested, tried, and sentenced the operators of the Drown Laboratories for "grand theft in diagnosing and treating patients for non-existent diseases with worthless electrical devices."[14]

Mechanical quacks have used gadgets with flashing lights, strange noises, dials and meters, and a multitude of electric wires under such names as Deploray, Electropad, Electron-O-Ray, and Ionic Charger. The last gadget was sold to treat rheumatism, insomnia, joint swelling, and skin diseases.

One gadget called the Voluptuizer was advertised as a bust developer to change a flat-chested girl into a girl with a full bosom. This gadget was sold through the mails. The Voluptuizer consisted of a plastic cup connected by a rubber tube to a rubber bulb (Fig. 1-3). The customer was instructed to apply a cream to the breast, clap the cup over the breast, and squeeze the bulb. The promoters sold $85,000 worth of

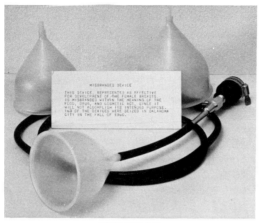

FIGURE 1-3
A misbranded plastic device that was promoted for the development of the female breasts. (Courtesy of the Food and Drug Administration, Dallas, Texas.)

Voluptuizers for $15 each. Other worthless gadgets have been sold by quacks to increase bust measurements.[15]

Many forms of gadgets and devices have been promoted to restore hair to balding scalps, correct sexual impotency, reduce pain of arthritis, increase the size of arm muscles, and reduce a person's weight. The mechanical quack, using some scientific-sounding title can put together a gadget or device to cure any disease, chronic health condition, injury, or mental illness. One gadget, for example, was merely an air-filtering mechanism in which a small fan pulled air through a filter in the back and past two small ultraviolet bulbs and then pushed it out again (Fig. 1-4). It was promoted for the relief of breathing difficulties, allergies, asthma, colds, sinus and hay fever.

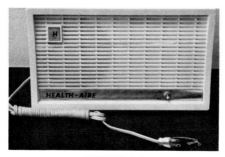

FIGURE 1-4
The Health-Aire, which was represented to create an atmosphere of "mountain air purity." (Courtesy of the Food and Drug Administration, Dallas, Texas.)

PSYCHOQUACKERY

Masquerading under a weird assortment of scientific titles, the psychoquack claims cures for mental illness, alcoholism, sexual inadequacy, and overweight. At least $375 million are earned each year by more than 25,000 psychoquacks in the United States. Occasionally, a psychoquack will have some preparation in psychology from one or two correspondence courses. Most psychoquacks are not licensed to practice psychiatry, psychoanalysis, or clinical psychology. Often psychoquacks have forged credentials or receive degrees from institutions with questionable reputations.

Most psychoquacks use sedatives and hypnosis, which can do serious harm to their customers. Without any consultation with a licensed medical doctor, the psychoquack starts his "treatments." The results are often tragic. Some patients have committed suicide; others have become permanent residents of mental hospitals.

Posing as a religion, Scientology has become a worldwide enterprise claiming to help mentally ill persons for sizable fees.[16] The promise of a quick and easy treatment for mental illness has led to tragedy and disaster for many victims of Scientology. Many persons with crippling diseases have been urged to join Scientology so that they can walk, work, or breathe without any crippling effects.

The founder of Scientology, L. Ronald Hubbard, has no college degree, even though Scientology literature indicates he has a B.S. in civil engineering and a Ph.D. and was "trained as one of the first nuclear physicists." Hubbard claims the mind is divided into two parts: analytical and reactive. The analytical mind is rational. It perceives things, reasons, and figures things out. The reactive mind takes over the analytical mind and causes unpredicatable behavior. The purpose of Scientology is to bring the reactive mind under complete control of the analytical mind. Thus, the person will overflow with happiness. When the person has reached this state of mind, the person is called, "clear." Hubbard claims the reactive mind stores "engrams"—impressions made by shock or pain on the mind. Another theory promoted by Hubbard is that each person has a "thetan" or spirit which is immortal and has lived within countless humans and animals. The thetan has numerous engrams. Each person must get rid of all engrams that his thetan has. When all engrams have been displaced, the person is "clear."

When the prospective member of Scientology enters into this cult, he is called a "preclear" encrusted with engrams. The member must pass through "grades of release" to get rid of his engrams. As the member proceeds from one "grade of release" to the next, he pays an exorbitant price to achieve "happiness." The preclear signs a contract for a series of sessions of one hour each with a Scientology "auditor." If the preclear completes the first four stages of release, he will pay about $1000.

One wealthy preclear spent $28,000 on the stages of release required of Scientology.

Upon entrance into Scientology, the preclear is controlled by the auditor's commands. Simple questions are answered and requests for certain actions are completed by the preclear. Then, the auditor asks oddly worded questions, some mind-numbing, for 25 to 75 hours. If a problem in the life of the preclear is mentioned by the preclear, the auditor turns away from the problem. The auditor pushes the preclear into a world of fantasy and uses a device called an "E-meter" to which are wires running to two tin cans held by the preclear. The auditor watches the E-meter's needle on a dial as the preclear answers. Movements of the needle indicate that the preclear is hiding some problem within his life. Eager to cooperate, the preclear accepts the auditor's statement that he is hiding some problem, even if he cannot remember what the problem is. The preclear believes he is experiencing engrams in his thetan's past. As the preclear reveals the engrams, he is told he is on the road to happiness. The preclear shows signs similar to those of schizophrenia. One preclear believed he was Marc Anthony and recalled Cleopatra but had no recollection of the battle of Philippi.

The Church of Scientology attempts to lure patients from psychotherapy. Scientology keeps the preclear in an illusory state for exorbitant fees. As the preclear drifts further from reality, he lives more and more in the world of Scientology. Converts of Scientology have been so deluded by the pseudoscientific jargon and rites that they believe only they know the truth and do not realize that they no longer can communicate with the rest of the world.[16]

WEIGHT-REDUCING QUACKERY

At least $2 billion to $10 billion is spent each year on diets, drugs, diet candies, slenderizing machines, quick-reducing gadgets, health spas, masseurs, and exercising machines by gullible customers to lose weight. Many Americans have tried steam baths as an instant way to reduce.

Obesity may be defined as the human body loaded with excessive fat. *Overweight* may be considered to mean in excess of the "average" weight.[17] Most obese adults have been fat children and teenagers. Preventing obesity in adulthood lies with changing children's eating patterns. Vigorous physical exercise, dietary education, and psychological support introduced into elementary and secondary school curricula can assist students to lose weight. Strenuous exercise in special physical education classes can be planned for the obese. Instruction concerning proper food intake can be given to obese children. Encouragement and motivation are examples of psychological support.[18]

Any weight-reducing program should be planned in cooperation with a medical doctor and a dietitian. Some hospitals have diet kitchens where the obese person can eat meals tailored to his caloric intake. His weight loss will be recorded, and his blood pressure and physical health will be checked by a physician. In addition, a record is kept of daily vigorous exercise.

Diets

So-called revolutionary weight-reduction diets have been introduced such as the high fat, high protein, banana, milk, grapefruit, DuPont, Rockefeller, Seven-day, Twelve-day, and "instant fat loss" diets. From March 1969 to February 1971, more than 70 diet articles appeared in popular women's magazines with such advice as "Dieting by Computer" and "Chewing Your Way to Health, Sexual Vitality, Peace." Advertised in newspapers and popular magazines, these diets are sold in printed form as a pamphlet, hardback, or paperback. These diets often require the customer to buy a "weight-reducing pill, tablet, wafer, liquid, food supplement, or special food." The "instant fat loss" diets are formula liquids or total daily diet products of 800 to 900 calories in a day. Some disadvantages of "instant fat loss" diets are gastrointestinal side effects and the possibility of omitting essential nutrients. Diets advertised may suggest starvation for a few days without any consultation with a physician or a water diet accompanied by one food.

Some advertised diets emphasize extensive use of grapefruit in combination with a low-carbohydrate, high-protein diet. This diet followed for many months without medical supervision can be harmful to persons with heart or kidney conditions.

One weight-reducing plan placed the person on a 500-calorie-per-day diet with regular injections of a hormone called human chorionic gonadotropin. The endocrinologist advocating this weight-reducing plan claimed that the hormone is involved with breaking up deposits of certain types of fat. No conclusive proof exists that this claim is true.[19]

Drugs

More than two billion diet pills are sold each year for weight reducing purposes. Gross sales are estimated from a quarter to a half billion dollars a year. Often sold without a physician's prescription or obtained from "pushers" of drugs and narcotics, these diet pills include drugs, prescribed and over-the-counter. Some of these drugs are amphetamines, diuretics, thyroxin, estrogen, digitalis, barbiturates, and laxatives. Without continuous medical supervision, any of these drugs used in combination or simply in overdose can be lethal. Since a large percentage of amphetamines and barbiturates are sold illegally, they can be obtained by weight-reducing quacks and sold to the customer. Amphetamines cause physical complications and barbiturates are addicting.[20] Amphetamines speed up activities of the central nervous system and suppress appetite. The person taking large amounts of amphetamines can reach a paranoid psychotic state. Barbiturates slow down activities of the central nervous system. The person taking increased amounts of barbiturates to counter the effects of amphetamines finds that sudden discontinuance of barbiturates can be extremely dangerous.

Indiscriminate use of other types of weight-reducing pills may be equally dangerous. Diuretics increase the production of urine from the kidneys. Thyroxin increases the rate by which the human body burns food. Estrogen may be in different forms of the female sex hormone. Digitalis is used for its effects upon the heart, but should not be used for weight reduction. Laxatives are mildly acting cathartics. Cathartics promote evacuation of the intestines. However, one person's laxative may be another's cathartic. Or, a laxative may be a laxative at one time and be a cathartic at another time in the same person.

The promoters of Anapex Diet Plan Tablets advertised that the tablets would help the user to lose "85 pounds of ugly fat in two short months." When these Anapex tablets were analyzed by a pharmacologist, they were found to contain benzocaine, methyl cellulose, thiamine mononitrate, sodium carboxyl methyl cellulose, and riboflavin. The dosage of benzocaine in the Anapex tablet had no anesthetic effect on the mucous membranes of the stomach or the intestinal tract to inhibit the person's desire for food. Methyl cellulose and sodium carboxyl methyl cellulose are "bulk producers" which enlarge within the stomach and diminish hunger contractions. Bulk producers have not been proven to change the physiological and psychological causes determining a person's appetite. Included along with the Anapex tablets was a modified high protein diet. However, the advertisement for the tablets stated that the diet was unnecessary.[21]

Bel-Doxin, another product removed from sales contained the drug scopolamine aminoxide. This drug produced drowsiness in its user so that the person reduced his food intake.[22]

Obesity-pill clinics, run for affluent obese customers, seldom permit the customers to meet or see the operator of the clinic. The operator, who calls himself "Dr ," contacts the customer by a tape recording and promises 15 to 30 pounds weight loss in the first month. Pills handed to the customer may be amphetamines, barbiturates, diuretics, or laxatives, or combinations of these drugs at a cost of $10. At the same time the attendant schedules another visit to the "clinic."

Diet Candies

The theory behind the diet-candy is that the candy raises the level of sugar in the blood before a meal, thus diminishing the appetite. Then, the person wishing to lose weight will have no trouble giving up foods high in calories. One brand of diet candy had 25 calories for each caramel. Directions on the box of caramels indicated two caramels had to be taken before meals. The 50 calories would be equivalent to about 3 teaspoonfuls of sugar. This amount of sugar has little effect on blood sugar levels.

Other diet candies often contain vitamin and mineral supplements. These supplements are not needed in the diet just because the diet is low in calories. A weight-reducing diet, low in calories, can contain proper amounts of vitamins and mineral elements. Green and yellow vegetables, skim milk, eggs, lean meat, fish, fowl, fruits, and some bread will contain the essential nutrients.

Slenderizing Machines

Either the customer buys the slenderizing machine for use in his home or he uses the machines in health clubs, gymnasiums, or slenderizing salons. These machines may reduce the waist measurement and not the weight. One manufacturer of these machines claimed his machine could stimulate muscles to contract by means of electrical impulses, thus improving muscle tone. The obese person's muscles were considered to be soft and flabby. Repeated use or contraction of a muscle should enlarge it.

Another slenderizing machine had a rhythmic, rocking motion which, according to the promoter, was equivalent to 36 holes of golf. This slenderizing machine, available for use in the home, was priced at several hundred dollars. Other slenderizing machines provided vibrations to parts of the human body. Promoters claim that their machines would produce a "graceful or handsome figure." through these vibrations. Some so-called slenderizing devices, such as mechanical rollers, can be operated by hand. Rolling the device over the hips is supposed to remove fat deposits under the skin.

One promoter of a slenderizing machine boasted that the machine could take inches off the waist. The machine was sold to 400,000 owners for $100 to $400 per machine and grossed the promoter $40 million. The Food and Drug Administration found that the machine would aggravate gastrointestinal, muscular, vascular, kidney, orthopedic, neurological, gynecological, and pelvic disorders of the owners (Fig. 1-5).

Quick-reducing Gadgets

Several millions of dollars have been spent by Americans for inflatable clothing, constricting bands and body suits, and weighted waist belts. One inflatable item was a plastic belt worn around the waist like an inflated inner tube. Inflatable shorts have been sold as "girth-reducing" shorts. The promoters guaranteed money refunded if inches were not taken off the girth. These inflatable types of clothing are supposed to create "hot spots" on the skin while exercising and thus shrink the skin. One promoter of inflatable clothing claimed the fatty deposits at the waist could move to another part of the human body.

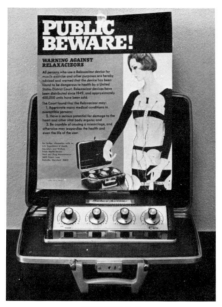

FIGURE 1-5

A weight-reducing device that provided vibrations to the body. (Courtesy of the Food and Drug Administration, Dallas, Texas.)

Constricting bands and body suits are advertised as "fat off" devices. The bands fit snugly around the thighs, upper arms, chin, and waist (Fig. 1-6). The promoters claim that the constricting bands squeeze fluid from the fatty tissue to other tissue of the human body. Also, the bands are to cause the obese to perspire and lose weight. The promoters claim that the body suits not only induce perspiration and sweat off

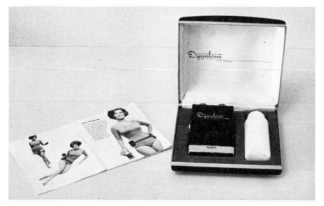

FIGURE 1-6

Constricting bands advertised for weight loss. (Courtesy of the Food and Drug Administration, Dallas, Texas.)

unwanted fat but also tone and massage the skin, even when the wearer is sleeping. Some body suits are plastic; others are nylon.

Weighted belts contain 10 to 15 pounds of steel or lead shot. The promoters claim the belts will cause the wearers to lose weight because of the added weight the wearers must carry. Also, the promoters advertise that the belts can "firm" the hips and thighs and be substituted for exercise. Other promoters have boasted that their weighted belts could whittle inches from the waist.

Exercising Machines

Americans spend at least $100 million on muscle stimulators and other exercising machines. The muscle stimulators are claimed to be effective in eliminating wrinkles and reducing weight. Their promoters advertise that the human body is bombarded with electrical charges by the stimulators, thus causing muscle contractions.

Spring platforms for jogging, unicycles, hand grippers, treadmills, stationary bicycles, and hundreds of other exercising machines are sold in the millions. Usually, the promoter does not tell his customer that the exercising machines must be used strenuously, daily, and for a long period of time. Instead, the customer relaxes and lets the machine pull him through the motions. The customer is deluded about the exercise that he is getting while using the exercising machine, for the promoter advertises that the exercising machine provides the same exercise as long-distance running or cycling.

Health Clubs, Spas, Salons

For a fee of $300 or more and a few visits a week, the customer is promised a quick weight-reducing or physical fitness plan in a health club, spa, or salon. Equipped with sauna baths, sun rooms, swimming pools, exercise areas, steam baths, whirlpool machines, vibrators, the clubs, spas, or salons offer the customer several free sessions along with his membership. The customer signs a contract with the owner. Calisthenics which build muscular strength are the traditional activities, in addition to the use of vibrating machines, steam baths, and exercise areas. Often persons in charge of the programs have no formal preparation in physical education and do not require the customer to have a medical examination before undertaking the exercise programs. Some of the exercises may be dangerous to the customer, particularly if the customer has injuries to lower back muscles, vertebrae, or knee joints or has some degree of atherosclerosis. The claims of the operators that exercises redistribute fat content, that passive vibrating equipment reduces weight, that the sauna baths reduce arthritis, acne, colds, or bronchial infections, or that whirlpools improve general health are false. The customer must pay the contracted price regardless of whether he acquires any beneficial results. In addition, the club, spa, or salon is absolved of responsibility for injuries incurred on its premises, such as strained muscles of the lower back. Claims of any health club, spa, or salon need to be carefully investigated before a contract is signed.[23]

OTHER TYPES OF QUACKERY

Unbelievable as it seems, quacks claim cures for male sexual impotency, epilepsy, diabetes, hearing deficiencies, alcoholism, kidney diseases, constipation, hemorrhoids, cerebral palsy, and heart diseases, to name a few. Nostrums or concoctions, gadgets, quick-cures, special diets, and devices discovered by quacks are available.

Quacks have exploited the age-old fears of male sexual impotency. It is estimated that the sales of pills, lotions, gadgets, and special treatments to improve sexual potency result in a multimillion dollar business each year. Advertisements for the product are usually mailed to adolescent boys and adult males and are worded in such a way that the product seems medically approved. Some of the ingredients in these products are concentrated horseradish powder, papaya leaves, food supplements, ground-up cockle burrs, buck shot, hot pepper, prickly ash bark, and mixtures of vitamin pills.

For the cure of epilepsy, the quack may give his customer drugs that should be taken only under medical supervision. One of these drugs is phenobarbital. The customer is attracted to the quack's advertisement of a miracle cure for epilepsy. The customer describes his condition which the quack pronounces as epilepsy. The quack has not relied upon the results of a medical examination, laboratory detection procedures, or the diagnosis of a medical doctor. In some cases, the customer does not visit the quack each month, since he needs only to send his money to the quack for the monthly supply of phenobarbital.

Some diabetics have become the victims of quacks claiming miracle treatments of diabetes without the injection of insulin, prescribed diet, exercise, or supervision of a medical doctor. Using diuretics and other worthless concoctions, the quack assures the diabetic that the miracle treatment can completely cure diabetes. One victim suffered diabetic acidosis or coma to such an extent that friends rushed the diabetic to the hospital. He had all the signs of diabetic acidosis or coma: nausea, vomiting, fruity breath, flushed and dry skin, deep and labored breathing, and drowsiness. Advice given by "health food" promoters, vitamin salesmen, and books written by nutrition quacks should be avoided by any person who has diabetes.

"Cures" for alcoholism, kidney diseases, hemorrhoids, and constipation are advertised by quacks. The customer buys a worthless tonic as a cure for his "liquor habits." The tonic may contain some vitamins, sugar, flavoring, water, baking soda, iron extract, and a pain reliever. Cures for alcoholism have been advertised by psychoquacks and naturopaths. Hypnotism may be prescribed by the psychoquack. Diuretics are common ingredients in "treatments" by quacks for kidney diseases. Sold for self-medication the treatment for kidney diseases may be advertised as the same treatment for bladder trouble. Many customers have bought cures to shrink hemorrhoids and to relieve itching and burning sensations accompanying hemorrhoids. Instead of consulting a medical doctor, the customer spends a small fortune on all types of cures for hemorrhoids. Many persons have attempted self-medication for constipation. Excessive and continuous use of laxatives not prescribed by a medical doctor may lead to colitis. Extremely dangerous too are experimentation with different laxatives and the use of an advertised high colonic enema without consultation with a medical doctor. The fallacy that "Each person must have a daily bowel movement" is commonly believed.

Many customers have bought concoctions for "tired blood" and self-diagnosed anemia. Countless advertised so-called cures for colds and coughs are sold as over-the-counter drugs to relieve the "miseries" of colds and coughs. Instructions on labels of over-the-counter drugs need to be read and carefully followed, particularly as to the dosage for children. Home remedies for colds and coughs should be avoided.

Some persons purchase eyeglasses, eye treatments, or hearing aids from door-to-door salesmen or by mail. The customer selects the eyeglasses from a variety of glasses without any consultation with an ophthalmologist or an optometrist. Or, the customer subscribes to a mail-order course in eye treatments to correct his vision defects. Hearing aids sold as cures of deafness often are costly and not suitable for the person with the hearing difficulties. Too often, the customer is totally unaware of conductive or perceptive deafness or that he can have a combination of conductive and perceptive deafness.

Quacks have offered many cures for high and low blood pressure. Some of these cures have been aspirin, laxatives, garlic, safflower oil, certain highly touted health foods, barbiturates, and antibiotics. So-called health foods are often falsely advertised to cure high (or low) blood pressure.

Other quack cures and treatments are for kidney trouble or painful urination. Cures for psoriasis are often available from quacks. As long as the exact causes of psoriasis are unknown, the so-called cures do not have any permanent effect. Not only are there many types of arthritis quackery but also cures for other aches and pains in the joints and muscles. Over-the-counter drugs as pain relievers provide temporary relief of pain. Persistent pain needs to be brought to the attention of a physician. Self-treatment for hernias is widely practiced by persons not understanding the need for medical care of hernias. All types of trusses or rupture devices can be purchased. Many pain relievers are purchased as a cure for sinus pain. Continuous, painful sinusitis needs the care of a medical doctor. The customer either tries to cure his ulcer by self-medication or buys a worthless nostrum from a quack. Ulcer cures can be extremely dangerous when the customer has signs of stomach cancer. Often the cure or treatment available from the quack is a secret remedy, advertised, and with a money-back guarantee.

In interviews with 2839 adults about their health practices and opinions, National Analysts found that many believed that personal health problems can be solved by trial and error, using questionable practices.[24]

1. Twelve percent of those interviewed reported they had arthritis, asthma, allergies, hemorrhoids, heart trouble, high blood pressure, and diabetes, even though these chronic conditions had never been diagnosed by a physician.
2. Twelve percent used self-medication without seeing a physician for sore throat, cough, insomnia, and digestive upsets.
3. Two percent indicated they "did something every day or nearly every day to help with bowel movements" and these actions were *not* taken upon a physician's advice.
4. Thirty-three percent followed fallacious concepts of weight control and 6 percent used questionable weight reduction practices.
5. Twenty percent had used something supposed to "cure" arthritis. Thirteen percent had tried something to "lubricate their joints"; 10 percent had tried vibrators; and 1 percent had worn brass or copper jewelry for their arthritis.
6. Twenty-five percent accepted cancer "cures" claimed by quacks.
7. One-half percent reported they had bought nonprescription (over-the-counter) medicine to help their hearing. These persons tended to be a younger age group. One percent purchased hearing aids that had not been prescribed by a physician.
8. Many persons engaged in questionable health practices by trial and error in the belief that "anything is worth a try" and it might work for them.
9. Greater-than-average acceptance of advertised claims existed for "tonic" use, weight reduction, and self-medication.
10. A substantial number of persons believed that advertisers in the health field are so rigorously regulated that serious distortions are unlikely.

The conclusion to be drawn from this study conducted for the Food and Drug Administration is that millions of Americans base important health decisions upon the chance that almost any treatment is beneficial, since individuals differ.

REFERENCES

1. Young, J. H.: The Medical Messiahs. Princeton, Princeton University Press, 1967, pp. 360-389.
2. American Cancer Society: Unproven Methods of Cancer Treatment. New York, The Society, 1966, pp. 53-73.
3. *Ibid.*, pp. 24-28, 38-39.
4. *Ibid.*, p. 41.

5. *Ibid.*, pp. 22-27, 28-29, 57-59, 72-74.
6. *Ibid.*, pp. 62-64.
7. *Ibid.*, pp. 47-49.
8. Young, *op. cit.*, pp. 316-332.
9. American Cancer Society: *op. cit.*, pp. 29-88.
10. Bruch, C. W.: Eye products: handle with care. FDA Consumer, 6:4, 1972.
11. "Paul Revere:" Dentistry and Its Victims. New York, St. Martin's Press, 1970, pp. 118-133, 239-241.
12. Kaplan, J.: Doctor Abrams—dean of machine quacks. Today's Health, 44:21, 1966.
13. Smith, R. L.: The incredible Drown case. Today's Health, 46:46, 1968.
14. Kaplan: *op. cit.*, p. 80.
15. Smith, R. L.: Mail-order doctoring—still a menace. Today's Health, 45:22, 1967.
16. Smith, R. L.: Scientology—menace to mental health. Today's Health, 46:34, 1968.
17. Mayer, J.: Overweight: Causes, Cost, and Control. Englewood Cliffs, New Jersey, Prentice-Hall, Inc., 1968, p. 28.
18. Seltzer, C. C., and Mayer, J.: An effective weight control program in a public school system. American Journal of Public Health, 60:679, 1970.
19. Singer, S.: When they start telling you it's easy to lose weight. Today's Health, 50: 47, 1972.
20. National Clearinghouse for Drug Abuse Information: A Federal Source Book: Answers to the Most Frequently Asked Questions About Drug Abuse (Revised). Rockville, Maryland, The Clearinghouse, 1971, pp. 17, 20.
21. Singer, S.: *op. cit.*
22. *Ibid.*
23. What you'd better know before joining a health club. Today's Health, 50:17, 1972.
24. National Analysts, Inc.: A Study of Health Practices and Opinions. Final Report. (Conducted for the Food and Drug Administration). Rockville, Maryland, FDA Press Office, 1972.

SUPPLEMENTAL READINGS

American Medical Association, Department of Investigation: Facts on Quacks: What You Should Know About Health Quackery. Chicago, The Association, 1967.
Better Business Bureau: Facts You Should Know About Health Quackery. Boston, The Bureau, 1967.
Editors of Consumer Reports: The Medicine Show. Revised edition. Mount Vernon, New York, Consumers Union, 1974.
Jones, K. L., Shainberg, L. W., and Byer, C. O.: Consumer Health, San Francisco, Canfield Press, 1971.
Kime, R. E.: Health: A Consumer's Dilemma. Belmont, California, Wadsworth Publishing Company, Inc., 1970.
Maple, E.: Magic, Medicine, and Quackery. London, Robert Hale, Ltd., 1968.
Seaver, J.: Fads, Myths, Quacks—and Your Health. New York, Public Affairs Committee, Inc., 1968.
Tuck, M., and Grodner, A.: Consumer Health. Dubuque, Iowa, Wm. C. Brown Company, 1972.

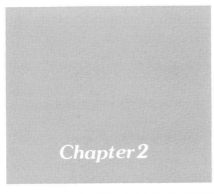

Chapter 2

FOOD FADDISM

AT least one billion dollars is spent on food faddism in one year. The number of stores specializing in food fads totals more than 3500. Chains of health food stores, as well as independently owned stores, are found in every state. Many major food chains have added "natural" food sections in their supermarkets. Food faddists sell all types of items: vitamin pills, books and pamphlets, concoctions, food supplements, utensils to prepare food, special diets to cure arthritis and other chronic health conditions, natural and organic foods in health food stores, and diet plans.

No age group is sufficiently informed about nutrition. More half-truths and misconceptions about nutrition are accepted by the American public than about any other type of health information, according to a report by National Analysts after interviews with 2839 adults.

1. Seventy-five percent believe that extra vitamins provide pep and energy.
2. Twenty percent indicated that arthritis and cancer are caused, at least in part, by deficiencies of mineral elements and vitamins.
3. More than half of the adults used vitamin pills without consultation with physicians.
4. Ten percent had eaten "organic, or natural food like health food stores sell." Nearly all health food users were acting without a physician's advice and expected to be "helped" by the health foods.
5. Health food users were more susceptible to testimonials in advertising and tended to rely on their judgment rather than that of a physician.
6. Twenty-six percent had used nutritional supplements without a physician's advice.
7. Seventy-five percent believed causes of poor health were more often due to "not eating right" than any other cause.

8. Many persons were convinced that one can "fine tune" his health by simply improving his diet.
9. For a majority of adults, food and nutrition become a likely route to "super" health.

The authors concluded that courses in schools with their stress upon general well-being rather upon specific diseases and chronic health conditions may contribute to the "super" health orientation.[1]

The National Nutrition Survey revealed more malnutrition in the United States than expected. Fifteen percent of all children in the survey showed evidence of growth retardation. Thirty-five to 55 percent of all children and adults had one or more deficiencies in their intake of required daily nutrients. Anemia was found among one third of the children and 13 percent of all age groups. Vitamin A deficiency was revealed in one third of all children. Among children from ages one to six years, 4 percent had a Vitamin D deficiency. Protein and calorie malnutrition was disclosed in 4 to 5 percent of all persons. Enlarged goiter was found among 5 percent of all age groups.[2]

WHAT IS NUTRITION AND WHAT ARE NUTRIENTS?

The science of food and its relation to health of all persons is nutrition. Chemical substances in foods are nutrients. They regulate body processes, repair cells, promote cell growth, and provide energy. The essential nutrients are carbohydrates, fats, proteins, vitamins, mineral elements, and water. Each food, such as milk, has some nutrients and falls within one of the Essential Four Food Groups (Table 2-1).

Carbohydrates

Carbohydrates are a major source of calories—the amount of energy (heat) required to raise the temperature of one kilogram (slightly over one quart) of water one degree centigrade. Carbohydrates consist of carbon, hydrogen, and oxygen. They add flavor to the menu and are economical. All carbohydrates are changed into simple sugars in the digestive process and provide energy for the human body. If there are excessive amounts of foods high in carbohydrates, the number of calories is increased. Common sources of carbohydrates are cakes, cookies, bread, dry cereals, granulated sugar, honey, preserves, dried fruits, potatoes, macaroni, rice, spaghetti, and grains such as wheat, rice, corn, and barley.

Fats

Fats are formed by the combination of fatty acids and glycerol. Fatty acids contain carbon and hydrogen with relatively small amounts of oxygen. Fats may be either solid or liquid at room temperature and will not dissolve in water. They provide heat and energy for the human body,

TABLE 2-1
ESSENTIAL FOUR FOOD GROUPS

Group	Daily Requirements	Equivalents
Breads and cereals	4 servings enriched, whole grain or restored breads and cereals, including enriched baked goods, macaroni, spaghetti, and noodles	1 slice bread = 1 serving ½-¾ cup cereal = 1 serving 1 cup enriched macaroni products = 1 serving
Milk and milk products	Children: 3 or more glasses Teenagers: 4 or more glasses Adults: 2 or more glasses	1 slice (1 oz) Cheddar cheese = ¾ cup whole milk ½ cup cottage cheese = ⅓ cup whole milk 2 tablespoons cream cheese = 1 tablespoon whole milk ½ cup vanilla ice cream = ⅓ cup whole milk
Vegetables and fruits	4 servings, including 1 serving citrus fruit or other source of vitamin C daily and dark green or deep yellow vegetable for vitamin A every other day	½ cup = 1 serving fresh, canned, or frozen fruit or vegetable
Meat and other protein foods	2 servings (meat, fish, poultry, eggs, beans, peas, lentils, nuts, or peanut butter)	1 oz cooked lean meat, poultry, or fish 1 egg ½ cup dried beans or peas 2 tablespoons peanut butter

help to regulate a person's body temperature, and insulate the body. Fats stored as fatty tissues within the human body may serve as a reserve of fuel. Support and protection of vital organs depend upon moderate deposits of fatty tissues. Polyunsaturated fats (vegetable oils and margarines) should be substituted for large amounts of animal fats. Common sources of fats are butter, margarine, vegetable oils, peanut butter, ice cream, meats and pork sausage, cakes, pies, cream, and whole milk cheese.

Proteins

Proteins contain nitrogen in addition to carbon, hydrogen, and oxygen. The structural units of proteins are amino acids which are essential for building and maintaining body tissues. At least 20 amino acids are known to be in proteins. A complete protein is one containing eight essential amino acids. Proteins furnish energy and promote repair, growth, and formation of new cells and tissues in the human body. Proteins regulate the water balance of the human body and the acid-base balance of the blood. This nutrient is not stored in large amounts within the human body. The sources of complete proteins are milk, eggs, meat, and fish. Incomplete proteins are derived from legumes, oatmeal, and root vegetables.

Water-soluble Vitamins

Vitamins are organic substances which usually are needed in small amounts to promote growth and maintain health. There are two types of vitamins in foods: water-soluble and fat-soluble. The water-soluble vitamins dissolve in heated water. They are excreted through the urine, and only small amounts are stored in the human body.

Ascorbic acid (vitamin C) helps to maintain firm healthy gums and aids in building and maintaining bones, blood vessels, and tissues. Vitamin C assists in maintenance of dentin of the teeth, helps to heal wounds, and helps to build resistance to infection. A daily supply of vitamin C is needed, since little of this vitamin can be stored. Some of the sources of vitamin C are oranges, lemons, grapefruits, tomatoes, strawberries, green leafy vegetables, cantaloupes, peppers, raw cabbage, and cauliflower.

Thiamin plays an important role in the life processes of individual cells of the human body. It promotes appetite and aids in assimilation and digestion of foods. Thiamin changes carbohydrates into energy and assists in building nerve stamina. Daily supplies of thiamin are needed, since only limited amounts can be stored in the human body. Some of the sources of thiamin are pork and other meats, fish, poultry, cereal products, dried beans and peas, nuts, and eggs.

Riboflavin assists in the metabolism (chemical changes) of carbohydrates, amino acids, and fats. It helps to maintain tissues of the skin, eyes, and nerves and promotes a feeling of vitality and well-being. Some of the sources of riboflavin are dairy products, meat, fish, poultry, eggs, cereal products, leafy vegetables, peas, and beans.

Niacin is necessary for growth and health of tissues. It promotes appetite, assists in the proper functioning of the digestive system, and helps to maintain healthy skin. Some sources of niacin are meat, fish, poultry, eggs, cereals, raisins, peanut butter, enriched bread, and dried peas and beans.

Fat-soluble Vitamins

Fat-soluble vitamins are absorbed from the intestines along with fats. They are insoluble in water. Fat-soluble vitamins are stored to a greater extent in the human body than are water-soluble vitamins. They are excreted.

Vitamin A is essential for growth, aids vision, and maintains epithelial tissues. It is essential for proper formation and maintenance of tooth enamel. Some sources of vitamin A are liver, egg yolk, dairy products, spinach, carrots, green and leafy vegetables, and apricots.

Vitamin D promotes growth and mineralization of bones and teeth. It improves the use of calcium and phosphorus within the human body and prevents rickets (a nutritional deficiency causing a weakening and enlargement of bones). Osteomalacia (a nutritional deficiency which results when bones are robbed of calcium, phosphorus, and vitamin D) does not occur if there is sufficient vitamin D. Some of the sources of vitamin D are egg yolk, butter, liver, fish liver oils, irradiated milk, and cream.

Mineral Elements

Mineral elements make up approximately 4 percent of a person's body weight. They serve as building materials and as body regulators. As building materials, mineral elements are essential in building bones and teeth. They assist in the formation of hair, nails, and skin. Muscles, glands, and nervous tissues need mineral elements as do the blood and the walls of arteries and veins. As body regulators, mineral elements regulate the exchange of body fluids and the movement of water in and out of tissues and assist in the control of glandular secretions. They maintain the normal irritability of nerve tissues and the contractility of muscle tissues. Mineral elements affect the clotting of the blood and oxidation processes.

Small amounts of mineral elements are needed in the daily diet. Calcium, phosphorus, and iron are often lacking. Iodine may be supplied through iodized salt and seafood.

Calcium is necessary for the formation and maintenance of bones and teeth. It is one of essential factors in blood clotting. Calcium, along with other mineral elements, is necessary for the rhythmic contraction and relaxation of the heart. Some of the foods containing calcium are milk and milk products, leafy and dark green vegetables, cereal products and beans, meat, fish, poultry, and eggs.

Phosphorus, which is often found in foods rich in proteins, is necessary for the formation and maintenance of bones and tissue. It is an essential part of every cell and tissue. Some of the foods containing phosphorus are meats, poultry, fish, eggs, cereal products, cheese, nuts, and milk.

Iron is essential in forming red corpuscles and hemoglobin (oxygen-carrying red pigment of the red blood corpuscles). Iron deficiency results in anemia, a condition in which there is a decrease in the quantity and/or quality of red blood cells. Some foods containing iron are meats, fish, poultry, eggs, cereal products, green leafy vegetables, dried peas and beans, dried fruits, and nuts.

Water

Water serves as a body regulator and as a tissue-building material. As a body regulator, water acts as a solvent. Cells must be kept in solution in order to maintain life processes and are three-fourths water. Water keeps substances in solution in gland secretions, in urine, and in circulating fluids. Water assists the flow of digestive juices and helps to dilute foods taken into the digestive system. It helps to regulate body temperature.

As a tissue-building material, water is the essential part of every kind of tissue. Bone is one-tenth water and blood is four-fifths water. Water is also necessary for tissue and bone maintenance.

Water loss can be replenished by including tap water, milk, and other beverages in the daily diet. Some foods, such as lettuce, contain 96 percent water.[3]

RECOMMENDED DAILY DIETARY ALLOWANCES

The basic nutrients—carbohydrates, fats, proteins, water-soluble vitamins, fat-soluble vitamins, mineral elements, and water—are needed each day by each person. The amount of nutrients and calories required varies by the age and sex of the person. Also, the recommended amount

TABLE 2-2
RECOMMENDED DAILY DIETARY ALLOWANCES*
NATIONAL ACADEMY OF SCIENCES, NATIONAL

	Age (years) from—up to	Weight kg	Weight lbs	Height cm	Height in	Energy Calories	Protein gm	Vitamin A activity (IU)	Vitamin D (IU)	Vitamin E activity (IU)
Infants	0.0—0.5	6	14	60	24	kg × 117	kg × 2.2†	1400	400	4
	0.5—1.0	9	20	71	28	kg × 108	kg × 2.0†	2000	400	5
Children	1—3	13	28	86	34	1300	23	2000	400	7
	4—6	20	44	110	44	1800	30	2500	400	9
	7—10	30	66	135	54	2400	36	3300	400	10
Males	11—14	44	97	158	63	2800	44	5000	400	12
	15—18	61	134	172	69	3000	54	5000	400	15
	19—22	67	147	172	69	3000	54	5000	400	15
	23—50	70	154	172	69	2700	56	5000	—	15
	51 +	70	154	172	69	2400	56	5000	—	15
Females	11—14	44	97	155	62	2400	44	4000	400	10
	15—18	54	119	162	65	2100	48	4000	400	11
	19—22	58	128	162	65	2100	46	4000	400	12
	23—50	58	128	162	65	2000	46	4000	—	12
	51 +	58	128	162	65	1800	46	4000	—	12
Pregnancy						+ 300	+ 30	5000	400	15
Lactation						+ 500	+ 20	6000	400	15

*The allowance levels are intended to cover individual variations among most normal persons as they live in the United States under usual environmental stresses. The recommended allowances can be attained with a variety of common foods, providing other nutrients for which human requirements have been less well defined.

†Assumes protein equivalent to human milk. For proteins not 100 percent utilized factors should be increased proportionally.

of nutrients is given in milligrams, grams, and international units, not in ounces and pounds. The accompanying chart has the recommended daily dietary allowances for practically all healthy people in the United States (Table 2-2).

WHY FOOD FADDISM EXISTS

Food faddism results when an incompetent person attempts to deal with nutrition of the human body. Since nutrition is basic to the well-functioning of the human body, it offers the widest possibilities for the promotion of products and misinformation. The vast number of myths and misconceptions about nutrition enables the faddist to operate without restraint. Food fallacies such as "fish is brain food," "white eggs are more nutritious than brown eggs," or "beets cleanse the blood" have been transplanted from the past.

Fear, superstition, gullibility, and hyponchondria have helped to pro-

TABLE 2-2
OF THE FOOD AND NUTRITION BOARD,
RESEARCH COUNCIL, REVISED 1973

Water-soluble vitamins							Minerals				
Ascorbic acid (mg)	Folacin* (µg)	Niacin† (mg)	Riboflavin (mg)	Thiamin (mg)	Vitamin B₆ (mg)	Vitamin B₁₂ (µg)	Calcium (mg)	Phosphorus (mg)	Iodine (mg)	Iron (mg)	Magnesium (mg)
35	50	5	0.4	0.3	0.3	0.3	360	240	35	10	60
35	50	8	0.6	0.5	0.4	0.3	540	400	45	15	70
40	100	9	0.8	0.7	0.6	1.0	800	800	60	15	150
40	200	12	1.1	0.9	0.9	1.5	800	800	80	10	200
40	300	16	1.2	1.2	1.2	2.0	800	800	110	10	250
45	400	18	1.5	1.4	1.6	3.0	1200	1200	130	18	350
45	400	20	1.8	1.5	1.8	3.0	1200	1200	150	18	400
45	400	20	1.8	1.5	2.0	3.0	800	800	140	10	350
45	400	18	1.6	1.4	2.0	3.0	800	800	130	10	350
45	400	16	1.5	1.2	2.0	3.0	800	800	110	10	350
45	400	16	1.3	1.2	1.6	3.0	1200	1200	115	18	300
45	400	14	1.4	1.1	2.0	3.0	1200	1200	115	18	300
45	400	14	1.4	1.1	2.0	3.0	800	800	100	18	300
45	400	13	1.2	1.0	2.0	3.0	800	800	100	18	300
45	400	12	1.1	1.0	2.0	3.0	800	800	80	10	300
60	800	+ 2	+ 0.3	+ 0.3	2.5	4.0	1200	1200	125	18+	450
60	600	+ 4	+ 0.5	+ 0.3	2.5	4.0	1200	1200	150	18	450

*The folacin allowances refer to dietary sources as determined by *Lactobacillus casei* assay. Pure forms of folacin may be effective in doses less than ¼ of the RDA.

†Niacin equivalents include dietary sources of the vitamin itself plus 1 mg equivalent for each 60 mg of dietary tryptophan.

mote the faddist. Despite scientific evidence concerning nutrition, the faddist appeals to the emotions of the consumer and not to the consumer's intelligence.

With our rapidly advancing technology that has devised new food products, the faddist can appear knowledgeable about nutrition. The person poorly informed about nutrition is confused by the new food products, especially when some faddists are promoting "back-to-nature" foods. Many customers of food faddism find it easier to accept the bizarre claims of the faddist than the valid facts of scientists in the field of nutrition. Too often, newspaper, magazine, and book publishers assume the claims of the faddist are authentic without checking with authorities in the field of nutrition.

The faddist has a diet or product for every disease, chronic health condition such as diabetes, injury, or mental illness. When medical science cannot give the patient an acceptable answer after diagnosis of some illness or injury, the faddist has the "cure" at a money-back guarantee.

Statements concerning nutrition made by physicians and other health services personnel may be misconstrued. Faddists take full advantage of these misconstrued statements. They may be supersalesmen distorting nutrition truths into pseudoinformation so that the customer cannot tell the difference between false information and scientific fact. The freedom of choice of many food products has permitted many Americans to become malnourished. The main ingredients in diets or products promoted by faddists include some "secret food or foods" to overcome this malnourishment or, as the faddist states, "nutritional bankruptcy."

The shortage of professionally trained nutritionists and dietitians increases the number of faddists. The *dietitian* specializes in serving food that is attractive, satisfying, and nutritionally adequate and organizes all phases of food production and service in an institution. A bachelor's degree in home economics with special emphasis on foods and nutrition plus additional graduate study and internship are usually required for this profession. A *nutritionist* is concerned with teaching the facts related to nutrition and with helping persons of different ages to get nutritious diets. Many nutritionists are employed by local and state health departments, other governmental agencies, and commercial groups. Other nutritionists teach in medical colleges and universities and are consultants to physicians and research workers. Not only a bachelor's degree in home economics with special emphasis on food and nutrition but also graduate study are required.

The inadequate number of personnel employed by official consumer protection agencies like the Food and Drug Administration and nonofficial protection agencies like the American Dietetic Association or the National Dairy Council makes the faddist secure in his promotion of nutritional nonsense, diet plans, and fraudulent products. Since the personnel of these official and nonofficial consumer protection agencies investigate and enforce legislation to protect the consumer, the faddist often does not come under their scrutiny because these agencies are understaffed and overworked.

NATIONAL HEALTH FEDERATION

Food faddists constitute the largest number of members of the National Health Federation purveyors of false health information and promoters of fraudulent products. Organized in 1955, the Federation has categories of membership ranging from $45 to $1000 a year. Established on a pyramid structure, the Federation permits ten or more persons to organize a local chapter and to receive a charter from the national office. The local chapter appoints one of its members to the County Health Federation which selects one of its members to the State Health Federation which, in turn, selects a member to the national organization. Members fall into two categories. In one category are the leaders of food faddism, quacks who have a national following, leaders of the health food movement, and leaders of the antifluoridation campaigns. In the second category are the converts of these faddists, quacks, and antifluoridationists. The monthly magazine of the Federation advocates worthless cancer treatments, mechanical quackery, antifluoridation, and nonsense from food faddists. The Federation has appeared before Congressional committees and conducts "postcard crusades" to influence state legislators. It condemns the Food and Drug Administration, the American Medical Association, the American Dietetic Association, the Postal Service, the Federal Trade Commission, and every reputable official and nonofficial consumer protection agency. Persons prominent as leaders in the Federation have been and are food faddists. One food faddist was convicted of misbranding more than 115 special dietary products for treatment of 500 diseases and chronic health conditions. Another was fined $6000 and sentenced to a year in prison for a dietary supplement which he claimed cured innumerable diseases. A food faddist and the Washington representative of the Federation promoted "dried Swiss whey" as an "intestinal tonic" and as a health food. Other leaders of the Federation operate chains of health food stores and sell vast quantities of fraudulent food products.[4]

CHARACTERISTICS OF THE FOOD FADDIST

Today's food faddist is a "food expert" with a pseudoscientific title and a booming business in miracle foods, dietary supplements, and other fraudulent products to promote "nutrition." With his health lectures and high-powered advertising he is much like the old-time medicine man who accompanied his sales pitch for quick cures with a vaudeville act in the town square.

The faddist has an overwhelming amount of zeal. An example is the vegetarian who eliminates all dairy and meat products from his daily diet and then seeks to convert others to his food fad. Another is the "natural food expert" who advocates that all foods should be grown without the use of commercial fertilizers and that commercially processed foods should be banned from the diet.

In public, the faddist will spout fallacies and half-truths to sell his products. In his home, he may eat a nutritious meal without including any of the products he sells. He laughs at the sucker who bought his product or products. Or, the faddist may be so firmly convinced that his fraudulent products are nutritionally sound that he limits his diet to these products until he becomes ill and needs hospital care.

The faddist is usually an attractive, a pleasant, poised, persuasive, and friendly person, who speaks and writes fluently. His products are often sold with a money-back guarantee. He may be an active member of the National Health Federation or some pseudoscientific organization.

Sales Techniques

The faddist has four techniques for reaching the public: (1) doorbell doctoring, (2) mail order, (3) "health" lectures and consultations, and (4) books and other printed materials. In the door-to-door doctoring, the faddist seeks entry into the customer's home where the faddist may make reckless and false claims about his products. Before being forced out of business by the Food and Drug Administration, one fraudulent food supplement producer employed over 50,000 door-to-door salesmen.

Faddists also contact prospective customers by advertisements sent through the mail. False and exaggerated claims for overpriced products are made and suggested methods for payment are described in the promotional materials. Usually an offer is made to refund the purchase price if the customer does not get the desired results.

Nutrition consultations by the faddist may take place in the customer's home, in the faddist's health food store or rented office facilities, or after a series of lectures in a rented auditorium. The faddist lends a sympathetic ear to the customer's ailments and has a product to sell after the "free" consultation. Since many people believe in the magical powers of food, the consultations provide a psychological lift so that customers forget their ailments.

Lecture series, advertised as "open" to the public, may deal with topics such as obesity, aging, diabetes, arthritis, cancer, sexual impotency, and beauty. The lecturer may advocate the use of health foods and promote his myths about nutrition and health. Often testimonials and claims for cures are used in promoting the products. The faddist may offer a book, pamphlet, or other printed material as inducements to have customers attend the lecture or buy the fraudulent products.

Today most bookstores offer a variety of publications by food faddists. One popular food faddist's book sold a half million copies, earning $250,000 in royalties for this author, almost one million dollars for book store owners, and a half million dollars for the publisher. Many reputable publishers have included food faddists' books in their lists.

One book, *Calories Don't Count,* written by a gynecologist-obstetrician, recommended a high fat, low calorie diet. Obesity was discussed, and readers were led to believe that the diet was a revolutionary reducing plan. The book was used to promote and sell worthless safflower oil capsules for treating obesity and atherosclerosis.[5] Another book, *Arthritis and Folk Medicine,* advised readers to prepare a mixture of honey and vinegar, with additional doses of kelp and iodine, as a treatment for arthritis.[6] *Good Health and Common Sense* advocated that the arthritic patient should avoid water at meals and drink cod-liver oil with orange juice.[7]

Considered the "High Priestess" of eating, Adele Davis was probably the most widely read author of questionable statements about nutrition. Miss Davis espoused the theory that most diseases, chronic health conditions, and other ailments may be due to some nutritional deficiency. Also, she claimed that every American suffers from nutritional deficiencies. Her books have appealed to college students, housewives, and the elderly. Many nutritionists concede that Miss Davis' interpretations of studies by authorities in nutrition and medicine are speculative, and they disagree with her recommendations for protein intake and extra-dietary supplements of vitamins D and A.

Lists of books written by food faddists can be obtained from the Council of Foods and Nutrition, the American Medical Association, and the Nutrition Foundation, Inc.

Diversity of Products

The faddist has a multitude of products or other items for sale. In addition to consultations, health lectures, and printed materials, faddists peddle health and organic foods, foods grown without pesticides and processed without food additives, hydroponically grown vegetables, food supplements, geriatric foods, Zen diet, overdoses of vitamin C, pills and capsules, "secret" remedies and concoctions, royal bee jelly, bottled water, and cooking utensils.

Health foods may be labeled as "organic," "unprocessed," "raw," or "natural." Special qualities of each health food are emphasized by the health food store owner. Some of these health foods and claims made by their producers are listed in Table 2-3.

TABLE 2-3
PRODUCTS PROMOTED BY FOOD FADDISTS

Products	Claims made by producers
Blackstrap molasses	Corrects baldness, aging, insomnia, and digestive disturbances
Carrot juice	Prevents varicose veins, gout, and Addison's disease
Honey and vinegar	Relieves constipation, decreases high blood pressure, cures diabetes; prevents asthma, tooth decay, inflammation of the kidneys, and corns
Ocean kelp	Provides pep and abundant health
Royal bee jelly	Prevents cataracts, alcoholism, and poorly developed muscles; restores sexual potency
Safflower oil	Prevents atherosclerosis and obesity
Wheat germ oil	Cures arthritis, prevents gallstones and cirrhosis, cures epilepsy, and prevents ulcers
Yeast	Rehabilitates worn body cells

Recently there have been increased sales of organic, unprocessed foods. Flour from grains such as barley, millet, and buckwheat has been promoted as superior to enriched white flour. Cranberry beans, sunflower seeds, black beans, red lentils, and unsulfured apricots have large sales. Health food store owners have advocated unleavened soaked-wheat bread which consists of corn oil, whole wheat flour, and whole wheat kernels, in addition to water and salt. Or, beverages may be of apricot milk, juices from unsweetened pineapples and raw cranberries, and honey and milk. Soups may be combinations of eggs, lemon juice, salt, and lamb broth. The food faddist suggests replacing table salt with sea salt, refined sugar with raw sugar, and pasteurized milk with unpasteurized milk. Most health foods sell for 30 to 100 percent more than the processed, inspected, and regulated food products.

Persons eating health foods have gone to great lengths to condemn the use of chemical fertilizers, pesticides, and food additives. According to the food faddist, chemicals in foods are the prime causes of our health problems. The faddist uses words like *toxic* and *poison* for foods that have been sprayed with pesticides or processed with food additives. He claims that pesticides are not needed because bugs can be picked off fruits and vegetables. Little does he consider that the cost of handpicking might make food so expensive that few persons could afford to eat. He scares the consumer by promoting the idea that all processed food is loaded with chemicals, and that many of these chemicals are toxic or carcinogenic. Often the faddist seems to overlook the fact that sanitary methods may not be followed in the preparation of health foods. He wants to return to the "good old days" when chalk was put in thin milk, peas were greened with copper, contaminated oysters were sold, lead and arsenic were added to baking powder, and decomposed beans were canned.[8]

The public readily accepts the food faddist's statements about the use of chemicals because the public does not understand their uses or the regulations controlling them. The faddist does not reveal that the amounts of pesticides and additives are miniscule traces and are closely regulated by the United States Department of Agriculture, the Environmental Protection Agency, and the Food and Drug Administration. Actually, all nutrients in foods are chemical substances.

Three studies of "organically grown crops" failed to show that these crops were superior to those grown under standard agricultural conditions with chemical fertilizers. (The shortest study lasted for 10 years, and the longest for 34 years.) Also, there is always the possibility of Salmonella contamination in organically grown health foods.

Pesticides include insecticides and must be used properly in spraying fruits and vegetables. The Food and Drug Administration sets limits on the amount of pesticide residue that may safely remain on fruits and vegetables at harvest. The consumer can protect himself further by thoroughly washing fruits and vegetables or by removing the skins.

A food *additive* is any substance intended for use in producing, preparing, packaging, transporting, or holding food. The classes of additives are nutrient supplements; nonnutritive sweeteners; preservatives; emulsifiers; stabilizers and thickeners; acids, alkalis, buffers, and neutralizing agents; flavoring agents; and bleaching agents. These additives have brought great improvement in the American food supply. The Food and Drug Administration has developed safety testing procedures and has devised methods for detecting and measuring additives in food. Once the additive is proved safe, the Food and Drug Administration issues a regulation which indicates a limit, or tolerance, in the amount to be used. If the additive is not proved safe or is misused, the processor has not complied with federal regulations.

Most nutritionists prefer to speak of "foods grown without the use of any fertilizers or pesticides and processed without the use of food additives or chemicals" rather than of "organically grown" foods. No federal agency or law defines and supervises the label "organic" and certifies that such foods do in fact fit that description. Legislation has been proposed to define "organically grown" foods, but such legislation would involve semiannual inspection of farms growing such foods and might indicate endorsement of them. Furthermore, no single food should be called "organic" because all foods are organic. No food should be labeled as a "health" food because all foods properly used in a nutritious diet benefit humans both physiologically and psychologically. No food should be termed "natural" because all foods are natural or are manufactured from natural foods.

Hydroponically grown vegetables are sold by some food faddists. These vegetables are grown indoors in water instead of in soil. Temperature and humidity are carefully controlled. Roots of the vegetables are fed a solution of organic, natural fertilizers. Vegetables grown by hydroponics have unusual quality, size, and nutritional value, but the prices charged are beyond the means of the average family's budget. Quality vegetables available at reasonable prices to all consumers contain the same nutrients as those found in hydroponically grown vegetables.

Food supplements have been advertised by the faddist to rid the customer of imaginary vitamin and mineral deficiencies which are claimed to cause ill health. The theory promoted by the producers of these supplements is that all diseases, disabilities, and mental illness are caused by malnutrition that can be corrected by using their products without any consultation with a medical doctor. These food supplements often far exceed the amounts of vitamins and mineral elements of the Food and Nutrition Board's Recommended Daily Dietary Allowances (Table 2-2). If the person includes the Essential Four Food Groups in his daily diet (Table 2-1), there is no need for self-dosing with food supplements.

The food faddist has developed a highly profitable market for geriatric foods. Promoted as meeting the special dietary needs of the elderly, these geriatric foods are expensive and unnecessary in the daily diet of the elderly. Usually the elderly have a reduced monthly income but believe they must buy these geriatric foods, even though they cost 30 to 100 percent more than foods of the Essential Four Food Groups. Actually, the nutritional needs of the older person are much like those of the average adult.

Some high school and college students have become infatuated with the Zen macrobiotic diet, a bogus version of the dietary discipline of Zen Buddhism. Recipe books and foods for Zen macrobiotic meals are found in the kitchens of many communes. Promoted by the late George Ohsawa, the Zen diet is claimed to prolong life. Its proponents believe that such foods as meat, fruit, and sugar stir up aggression in man and make him cruel and violent. In the Zen diet, there are 10 stages. The first stage includes chicken, vegetables, fruit, seafoods, cereals, and a lot of brown rice. Each successive stage reduces the variety of foods until the only food is brown rice. Water and other liquids, except tea, are drastically restricted. Ohsawa also excluded coffee, most spices, yeast, and chemically fertilized vegetables. The Zen faddist must have a spoonful of sesame salt in the daily diet. Actually, the Zen Buddhists include the foods excluded by the faddist of the Zen diet.

The Ohsawa Foundation advertised fraudulent medical claims. Such items as Japanese pumpkin and dragon tea were sold as cures for diabetes, kidney disease, morning sickness, and asthma. In addition, the Zen diet has been advocated as a way to lose weight. It could cause death if the person stayed on the diet for more than eight months. In one grand jury investigation into the death of a Zen diet faddist, it was revealed that a few months on the Zen diet had produced scurvy that had resulted in the death of the faddist.

Many food faddists advocate large quantities of vitamin C to cure common colds and other ailments, including cancer. These claims are based upon published reports of Nobel laureate Linus Pauling, who suggests that the ascorbic acid vitamin "may play a role in cancer control by strengthening tissues and therefore, could be effective in preventing the infiltration of those tissues by malignant cells in the body."[9] Pauling's paper on the therapeutic implications of vitamin C was rejected by the National Academy of Sciences. The amount of vitamin C prescribed by Pauling is from 250 to 10,000 milligrams (10 grams) as a preventive and from 1 to 15 grams a day as therapy for a cold. This prescribed amount is 4 to 250 times the amount for adults in the Food and Nutrition Board's Recommended Daily Dietary Allowances. With the ingestion of 4 or more grams of vitamin C daily, frequency of kidney stones may be increased in persons disposed to gout. Large amounts of vitamin C in the urine may interfere with testing the urine for sugar. Excessive intake of vitamin C during pregnancy may result in scurvy in infants who have a normal intake of vitamin C after birth.[10]

Pills and capsules are often sold door-to-door as food supplements. One food supplement was advertised as having 94 ingredients in its capsules and was suggested as a cure for cancer, muscular dystrophy, arthritis, cardiovascular diseases, aging, and sterility. According to the label for another food supplement, the pills contained unsaturated fatty acids, alfalfa juice, bioflavonid complex, and various mineral and trace elements for human nutrition. The Food and Drug Administration claimed that these capsules and pills were labeled incorrectly and that the mineral content was less than the amounts specified on the label.[11]

"Secret" remedies and concoctions have been promoted by other food faddists. "Natural" celery juice was proposed as a part of the therapy for hypertension, arthritis, neuritis, chronic appendicitis, and atherosclerosis. Faddists' teas, brews, and tonics have been advertised as cures for epilepsy, cataracts, kidney stones, varicose veins, and arthritis. Faddists have suggested using their recipes of mineral oil instead of salad dressing. One faddist's concoction was composed of 18 ingredients from corn syrup to powdered carrots. Another concoction included water cress, mint leaves, buckwheat, parsley, alfalfa, wheat germ, prunes, egg shells, and yeast. "Secret" remedies may consist of a variety of herbs packaged for curing many diseases and ailments.

Sea and ocean waters have been promoted by faddists to prevent aging and to cure arthritis, diabetes, multiple sclerosis, leukemia, cancer, and Parkinson's disease. "Natural" salt has been advertised to prevent calcium deposits in the joints.

"Immune milk" has been a favorite fraudulent product promoted by faddists. "Immune" milk is advertised to come from cows injected with "vaccines" containing streptococci and staphylococci.

Royal bee jelly has been promoted by both the cosmetic quack and the food faddist. One faddist claimed that an ounce of royal bee jelly, at $140, was an excellent source of vitamin B. The amount of vitamin B—thiamin, riboflavin, and niacin—recommended by the National Research Council's Recommended Daily Dietary Allowances is readily available in the Essential Four Food Groups at far less cost.

Sales of bottled water have enriched the bottlers by millions of dollars. Home sales of bottled water have risen by 50 percent and increase at a rate of 10 percent annually. At least 150 million gallons of water are sold as bottled water each year. The words, "sparkling," "natural springs," "scintillating," and "clear" are used in advertising. In an investigation of one bottler's product, it was found that 100,000 bacteria per liter were in the bottled water. The bottled water may be the same as the customer's tap water, since only half the bottled water sold comes from underground springs.[12]

Food faddists have also advanced the theory that certain types of cooking utensils are harmful to foods. Two fallacies are: aluminum cooking utensils cause cancer and Teflon-coated utensils are dangerous. The faddist has a full supply of his cooking utensils, at an exorbitant price, to take the place of aluminum and Teflon-coated utensils which have undergone careful testing by the manufacturer and the Food and Drug Administration.

MYTHS PROMOTED BY FADDISTS

To sell their diversity of products, faddists promote many myths. Some of these myths are: (1) vitamins should be taken for nutritional insurance; (2) most diseases are due to improper diet; (3) soil depletion causes malnutrition; (4) chemical fertilizers poison the land and crops grown on the land; (5) certain foods possess magical powers; (6) commercially processed foods are not nutritious; and (7) subclinical deficiencies are constant dangers.

The food faddist advocates that nutritional insurance provides the differences between robust health and illness. To get the nutritional insurance, the customer must take excessive amounts of vitamins sold by the faddist. Scientific evidence indicates that excessive quantities of vitamins administered artificially are excreted in the urine. If the person has an inadequate daily intake of vitamins, his capacity for storage of excess vitamins may be impaired. Fortunately, most vitamins are nontoxic so that excessive doses of self-prescribed vitamins do not bring serious consequences. However, there is evidence that excessive amounts of vitamin D daily over a long period may do harm. The Council on Foods and Nutrition, American Medical Association, has indicated that escessive amounts of vitamin D for a period of several months slows growth, decreases appetite, and reduces the total retention of calcium and phosphorus. Some faddists claim that extra vitamins will prevent or lessen the effects of infectious diseases. Vitamin C is the vitamin most often associated with this myth.

Vitamin E has been enthusiastically promoted by the food faddist as a preventive, a treatment, or a cure for the following:

angina pectoris	bee stings
arteriosclerosis	diaper rash
blood clots	frostbite
congenital heart disease	radiation burns
heart attack	skin burns
varicose veins	
	acne
arthritis	Buerger's disease
asthma	bursitis
crossed eyes	jaundice
cystic fibrosis	
detached retina	chronic constipation
diabetes	emphysema
hemophilia	poor posture
muscular dystrophy	
myasthenia gravis	labor pain
strokes	low sperm count
ulcers	miscarriage
	sterility

Faddists claim that millions of Americans whose intake of polyunsaturated fats is low must take vitamin E supplements. The National Research Council in its Recommended Daily Dietary Allowances set 12 to 15 international units of vitamin E per day for adults and indicated that the adult with 10 or less international units of vitamin E had sufficient vitamin E. The faddists have claimed vitamin E protects humans from air pollution. These claims were based upon experiments with rats particularly vulnerable to ozone or nitrogen dioxide toxicity. The faddists have touted the need for 10 to 20 times the amount of vitamin E recommended by the National Research Council for arteriosclerosis, hypertension, rheumatic heart disease, old and new coronary heart disease, and angina pectoris. More than 20 years ago, the worthlessness of vitamin E for the treatment of heart disease was reported in medical journals. Today, most cardiologists and medical researchers indicate that vitamin E has no value in the treatment of heart disease. The evidence that vitamin E might be useful in the treatment of intermittent claudication—a vascular condition in which the lower limbs receive less circulation of blood and the patient has pain when walking, particularly in the calves—is inconclusive.[13]

The myth that all diseases are due to improper diet is a favorite topic of the faddist. He overlooks the scientific evidence that many diseases are caused by bacteria, viruses, fungi, protozoa, helminths or metazoa, and rickettsiae. He suggests that diseases are due to chemical imbalances of a faulty diet. Thus, the faddist has a product, with a long list of ingredients, to prevent the chemical imbalance by providing the necessary ingredients lacking in the diet.

One argument used to sell food supplements is that soil depletion causes malnutrition. This myth implies that soil in the United States has become impoverished because of repeated tilling of the soil. Thus, the crops from this soil are deficient in vitamins and mineral elements. There is no scientific evidence that the nutritive values of crops have decreased with repeated tilling of the soil. The quantity of crops has increased with the use of fertilizers. Actually, foods grown on the "depleted" soil are providing more than enough of every nutrient needed by humans.

Some faddists promote the myth that chemical fertilizers poison the land and crops grown on the land. These faddists would have the public return to the raw, unprocessed, or natural foods raised without fertilizers. There is no scientific evidence that chemical fertilizers poison the crops, particularly when the fertilizers are used properly. If composting (reduction of systematically layered organic waste material to a rich humus) was used, the amount of compost needed to fertilize the usual size of vegetable field would be beyond the vegetable producer's capacity to handle.

The magical powers of certain foods are also a favorite theme of faddists. These foods have wonderous powers to protect the human from all types of diseases. The faddist has promoted the sales of whole grain flour, bread, cereals, raw fruits and vegetables, and foods sweetened only with honey or blackstrap molasses. Yogurt, a fermented milk product from whole milk, is another food highly "advertised" by faddists.[14]

The faddist advocates that commercially processed foods are not nutritious. In fact, processing of food is essential to its preservation, appearance, storage, and safe delivery. Modern food processing restores nutrients such as vitamin B and iron lost in the milling of white flour. Pasteurization of milk kills pathogenic bacteria causing diseases in humans. Vitamins and mineral elements have been added to oleomargarine and bread in the processing. With the addition of these nutrients in the processing of foods, the incidence of nutritional deficiencies such as rickets and pellagra is less than it was 50 years ago. The amounts of protein, iron, vitamin A, thiamin, riboflavin, niacin, and ascorbic acid in commercially processed foods have slightly exceeded the amounts needed per capita.

"That tired feeling" or those aches and pain are the results of a subclinical deficiency, so say the food faddists. The subclinical deficiency has been defined by the faddist as a deficiency not observable but suspected. Despite the lack of evidence that aches, pains, and "tired feeling" are due to vitamin deficiency, the faddist offers a supply of vitamin pills to cure the subclinical deficiency. In one well-controlled scientific study, supplements of vitamin B given to healthy persons, with an adequate nutritious diet, did not reduce the incidence of minor illnesses and did not produce a sense of unusual well-being.

Lack of scientific information about nutrition makes the consumer a prey to these myths about food and nutrition. The food faddist prospers because he claims his fortified, restored, enriched, energy-producing, low calorie, low sugar, low salt, low fat, and/or high protein products will enable the buyer to have a healthy, robust life. Knowledge of the facts about nutrition is the consumer's protection against the faddist.

REFERENCES

1. National Analysts, Inc.: A Study of Health Practices and Opinions. Final Report. (Conducted for the Food and Drug Administration). Rockville, Maryland, FDA Press Office, 1972.
2. Loyd, F. G.: Finally, facts on malnutrition in the United States." Today's Health, 47:32, 1969.
3. Guthrie, H.: Introductory Nutrition. 2nd Edition. St. Louis, Missouri, C. V. Mosby Co., 1971, pp. 20-276.
4. Smith, R. L.: Amazing facts about a 'Crusade' that can hurt your health. Today's Health, 44:31, 1966.
5. Taller, H.: Calories Don't Count. New York, Simon & Schuster, Inc., 1961.
6. Jarvis, D. C.: Arthritis and Folk Medicine. New York, Holt, Rinehart, & Winston, Inc., 1960.

7. Alexander, D. D.: Good Health and Common Sense. New York, Crown Publishers, Inc., 1960.
8. Deutsch, R.: Where you should be shopping for your shopping. Today's Health, 50:16, 1972.
9. Academy turns down a Pauling paper. Science, 177:409, 1972.
10. Vitamin C, Linus Pauling and the common cold. Consumer Reports, 36:113, 1971.
11. Proceedings of the Second National Congress on Medical Quackery, Chicago, American Medical Association and the Food and Drug Administration, 1963, p. 11.
12. Ferris, J.: Pure, scintillating, refreshing mountain spring bottled water anyone. Today's Health, 50:54, 1972.
13. Vitamin E. Consumer Reports, 38:10, 1973.
14. Bogert, L. J., Bragg, G. M., and Calloway, D. H.: Nutrition and Physical Fitness. 8th Edition. Philadelphia, W. B. Saunders Company, 1966, p. 326.

SUPPLEMENTAL READINGS

Bauer, W. W.: Potions, Remedies, and Old Wives Tales. New York, Doubleday & Company, Inc., 1969.
Better Business Bureau: Consumer's Buying Guide. New York, Rutledge Books, Inc., 1969.
Deutsch, R.: Nutritional nonsense and food fanatics. Proceedings, Third National Congress on Medical Quackery. Chicago, American Medical Association, 1966.
Fletcher, L. K.: An Investigation of Nutrition Quackery, 1960—. Unpublished Master's Thesis, The University of Texas at Austin, 1969.
Kime, R. E.: Health: A Consumer's Dilemma. Belmont, California, Wadsworth Publishing Company, Inc., 1970.
Margolius, S.: The Innocent Consumer vs. The Exploiters. New York, Trident Press, 1968.
Margolius, S.: Health Foods: Factors and Fakes. New York, Walker & Company, 1973.
Schoenfeld, D., and Natella, A. A.: The Consumer and His Dollar. Dobbs Ferry, New York, Oceana Publications, Inc., 1966.
Tatkon, M. D.: The Great Vitamin Hoax. New York, Macmillan Company, 1968.
Tuck, M., and Grodner, A.: Consumer Health. Dubuque, Iowa, William C. Brown Company, 1972.
Young, J. H.: The Medical Messiahs. Princeton, Princeton University Press, 1967.

Chapter 3

CULTS AND FALLACIES

WHILE man has traveled in space and walked upon the moon, some young adults in the most advanced and developed nations practice witchcraft. Others accept the treatment of diseases by traiteuses, powwowers, root doctors, and curanderas. At the same time, more and more investigations have revealed the influence of folklore and folk medicine, family and social customs, and health fallacies of ethnic groups upon health practices.

For many, the cults have special reasons for their existence. These cults may be the person's means of escaping the realities of everyday life, defying authorities, enforcing self-identities, satisfying unacceptable sexual behavior, using narcotics and hallucinogens, and adhering to diets nutritionally unsound

WITCHCRAFT

Today, more than 400 witch covens exist in the United States, with more than 150,000 members. A coven is a circle of 13 witches, mainly women, sometimes with a few men. Each coven has a Grand Master who is always a male and may be the devil. The coven meetings are attended regularly, and a grand meeting is held at the end of each quarter. Maiden, Dame, Devil-God are some of the names used in a coven of which several covens may be in one area of a community.

As early as 3000 B.C., amulets and talismans were common among the Babylonians, Egyptians, Phoenicians, and Abyssinians. Amulets, as well as witchcraft, were also common in medieval Europe. An amulet could be an object that preserved man from some trouble, a substance used in treating the ill person, or a treatment used to prevent illnesses. The talisman was intended to perform a specific task and could be placed on the ground with money or treasure.

Witchcraft may be a body of beliefs having to do with health and sickness and using a deified herd animal such as a goat, half human and half bestial, which appeared as Dionysus or Bacchus. Witchcraft may be the practice of white magic, consisting of charms or spells used for benevolent purposes, e.g., carrying a rabbit's foot or placing a horseshoe over a doorway. Witchcraft may be black magic where magic is used maliciously, calling upon the Prince of Evil to accomplish the evil. Or, the witch may no longer merely be invoking the devil's aid through her charms and spells but has made a contract to serve the devil. Charms could be drugs like belladonna or hair and nails of a victim. Victims of witchcraft suffer from hallucinations, hysteria, self-injury, and skin lesions. Covens have their own *Book of Shadows*—a collection of their established routines and ceremonials. The symbol of witchcraft is the pentagram or a five-pointed star drawn inside a one-foot circle and placed in the center of the altar. Witches' power is a highly organized, concentrated surge of thought energy being transmitted in a clear-cut and planned manner. At the coven, there may be ritual dancing, chanting, exhilaration, and thought-directed and highly disciplined performances intended to "burn" out the diseases area of a human. As soon as the human recovers from the illness, the ill person's own electromagnetic field is "straightening out" the diseased area. Herbs and potions are used, as well as charms, amulets, and talismans.[1]

Other charms used in witchcraft are full moon ring, Isis full-morning (Isis—ancient goddess of the full-moon ring moon) blood charm—few drops of blood, love tea, spice rubbed over the lover's body to increase sexual activity, colored candles, spells of all types including self-hypnosis, and the Cleopterous charm which was intended to insure satisfying love life and increase sexual vitality. Witchcraft is rich in ritual.[2] The language of a coven is poetic.

OBEAH, MACUMBA, VOODOO

Other forms of sorcery and magic ritual are obeah, macumba, and voodoo which were brought to the Western Hemisphere by African slaves. Many of the beliefs are still practiced today. Among the blacks of the British West Indies, the Guianas, and the United States, conjurer women are witches who use *obeah* as the power of the witch for good or evil. In Brazil, a cult similar to obeah is *macumba*, a mixture of Christian and pagan beliefs. The rites of macumba take place on January 20, the feast day of St. Sebastian, when participants dance to throbbing drums. Persons achieving a trancelike state convey to others the wisdom of the gods.

Voodoo, which derives from African ancestor worship, is practiced in Haiti and in the United States. Voodoo, also known as *VOO DOO, voudow, voudu, vodoo, voodu, vudu, and Hoodoo* is believed to permeate Haitian society today. The supernatural is invoked to teach young children to believe, to cure illness, and to curse enemies. The gods or spirits are known as "loa." The living corpse is the body from which the soul has been taken and is called the zombie. The body, called the "corps cadavre," has two souls.[3]

The area in the United States most affected by voodoo has been and is southern Louisiana. The most powerful figures among blacks of New Orleans were voodoo queens who presided over ceremonial rites. Voodoo doctors occupied secondary positions in the voodoo hierarchy. Voodoo queens and doctors were practitioners of black magic and had large incomes from selling charms, magical powders, and amulets—all guaranteed to cure the purchaser's every illness, grant his desires, and destroy his enemies. The voodoo queen or doctor would show her or his powers by having a rooster tied to a tree, plucked of every feather, and stuck with 9 silver pins in its breast. Or, the rooster would be dressed in a coat, trousers, and a hat. Or, a plate of "congris"— black eyed peas and rice cooked with sugar—would rest on dewy grass under a sycamore tree surrounded by a ring of silver coins. Or, hoodoo people could put poison in the drink or food of an enemy.

Some of the beliefs of voodoo still found in southern Louisiana concern the traiteur (man) and traiteuse (women). These are nonmedical people who treat ailments and disease. Traiteurs wet fingers with spit, trace a cross on the sick part of the human, make a sign of the cross, and say certain words or prayers. Traiteurs treat angina, erysipelas, rheumatism, tumors, arthritis, and dislocations. They prescribe a novena and apply an ointment or lotion such as dew gathered in the month of May. For chest ailment, the traiteuse rubs the patient's chest with Mentholatum on yellow cotton and hits "the wall with flat of hand three times." For rheumatism, the traiteuse mixes Black Diamond tobacco, salt, and kerosene together and says the Lord's prayer. Often, the traiteuse uses string with nine knots in it, which she ties while saying a prayer. The nine knots in the string represent the nine disciples. Often, ignorant folk have more faith in conjuring than in medical treatment. They believe an illness to be half-cured if pain is alleviated. If the illness is not cured, the cause may be attributed to delay in assisting the traiteur.

The following practices were found among certain ethnic groups in southern Louisiana in 1970:

1. For treatment of asthma
   a. Have a Chihuahua dog as a household pet.
   b. Catch a fish, breathe into its mouth. Before the fish's last breath, throw it back into water.
   c. Give the person with asthma a teaspoon of bluing.
   d. Place a knotted string tied around neck of the person with asthma and say prayers over knots as they are tied.

2. For treatment of syphilis
   a. Burn corn, put it in water, let it settle, have the infected person drink the water.
   b. Sleep with a virgin.
3. For treatment of rheumatism
   a. Wear a string with knots around part of body having rheumatism.
   b. Split a frog, fry in hog lard, rub on part having rheumatism.
   c. Tie a string with twelve knots around the neck.
4. For relief from labor pains
   a. Put scissors under bed to cut pain.
   b. Place a knife under mattress.
5. For treatment of infant who is teething
   a. Dry and string swamp lily root around baby's neck.
   b. Place a dried pumpkin stem on a string around baby's neck.
6. To offset discomfort or colic in a new infant from a visit of a menstruating woman
   a. Tie a black string around baby's waist.
   b. Tie black thread with nine knots around baby's wrist.
   c. Obtain a pin from the menstruating woman and pin it on the baby's clothing.
7. For treatment of whooping cough
   a. Give tea made from sheep manure.
   b. Pass child with whooping cough through a horse's collar which must be warm and damp from horse's sweat.
8. For treatment of diarrhea
   a. Tie a string with knots around the neck.
9. For a crooked neck
   a. Wear a black thread with three or four knots in it.
10. For treatment during menstrual period
    a. Tie a string with nine knots around the waist.
11. For a large navel
    a. Wear a string with eight knots around the waist.
12. For casting a spell to hurt a person or cause illness
    a. Take menstrual "pieces" and they will "drive a person crazy."
    b. Spill something on the floor; the person, to be affected, walks over the spill; person has pains in legs and has difficulty in walking.
    c. Place a small bag with dried bones, fingernails, and a chicken eye under the affected person's pillow to drive the affected person insane.
13. For warding off evil spirits
    a. Use bag with black cat bones, a bag with good smelling powder, or a bag with rat and hog bones, teeth, and dog hair.[4]

Gibbs cites a modern voodoo belief to correct a deformity. The person is instructed to find a four-leaf clover in a green pasture and get the wishbone of a chicken. Then he must get a bucket of fresh spring water and add the leaf and bone to it. Next, the person must remove all his clothes and look at the deformed part of his body through the reflection of the water until he is tired. Then the person pours the water over his entire naked body and lies under an oak tree in a forest and goes to sleep. When the person awakens, his deformity will have evaporated with the evaporation of the spring water.[5]

ROOT DOCTOR

From Wilmington, North Carolina, to Miami, in cities like Charleston and Savannah, in the Low Country (marshy sea islands along the Carolinas and Georgia coastline), and inland such as Beaufort County, South Carolina, the root doctor can be found placing a "root" or spell upon humans. This practice was also brought by African slaves to the American colonies. Many large cities have at least one store where the do-it-yourself believer in root can buy the "root."

Today, the root doctor deals with autosuggestion in an individual's subconscious mind. The root doctor uses tokens or charms, called "roots," of varying colors and powders. These tokens are not used as curatives but are hidden near the "hexed" person for the "hoped-for-effect." A token of one color is supposed to cast a spell, but another token of another color or another color of the same token is reputed to remove the spell or root. The tokens or charms have been made of flannel and shaped like a carrot. Threads like a small root protrude from the pointed end. Charms have secret ingredients—dirt from a graveyard taken at midnight, the heart of an owl, frog's feet, or crushed bone. The root or charm is sewed inside clothing and usually costs $100. Roots come in three colors: (1) red for sickness or death, (2) blue for protection against evil and help in love affairs, and (3) black for money. The root's power increases in direct proportion to the size of the client's pocketbook.

The root doctor is sought when a person believes he has been wronged by someone, his luck has been unduly bad, or someone has put a root on him. The root doctor is a firm believer in his powers. The "Doctor" will let the hexed person talk, listen to the person, and make "root" to help the person. The office of the root doctor might be filled with mysterious, stuffed animals and birds, potions, and medicine bottles. The root doctor wears dark glasses and speaks in an "unknown tongue" as he prepares the root. Mystery surrounds the preparation of the root. Seldom is there a dissatisfied customer because if the root fails, the person receiving the root is to blame.

In one instance, a divining root switch, used by the root doctor, made a "hexed" sick woman rise out of bed and find the root buried in the ground. The divining root switch found the buried root. The root doctor tore the root from the ground. The ill woman recovered from her illness.

Not only charms like dirt are used but also a guinea hen feather, small bone, and sulphur—all placed in a glass jar—are called the "root." Root powder is sold in tobacco sacks. It is believed that the powder has root and can be poured on the ground in the shape of a cross. If an enemy walks across the cross, he may never walk again.[6]

Dr. Ramsey Mellette, Jr., Director, Child Psychiatry Unit, Medical University of South Carolina, Charleston, has indicated that autosuggestion from a root doctor can be so overpowering that the "hexed" victim is unable to think of anything else.[7] The hex or root can cause good or evil, weakness, suffering, confusion, misery, pain, impotence, sickness, and death. The "white" or good root can produce success, recovery from illness, and protection against bad roots. Persons living in parts of New

Jersey have a root which consists of "real 'bad news' kind." Many large cities have at least one store where the do-it-yourself believer in root can buy the root equivalent, in a concoction made by a quack.

The root doctor does not dispense medication illegally, uses no oral cures, and sells root bags and mystical powder. When the root doctor "chews the root," he is actually chewing on a piece of root. When the root is chewed during a court trial, the root doctor is attempting to render evidence harmless, thus influencing the outcome of the trial. To counteract a patient's hex from a root doctor, medical doctors, after all other medical treatments have failed on a patient, may use a placebo, nicotinic acid, or calcium gluconate to "burn" the "hex" out of patient.[8]

HEX SIGNS AND POWWOWING

Geometric designs or *hex signs* on the big red barns of southeastern Pennsylvania have been topics of widespread interest. Some believe that the six-pointed star painted on a barn protected the barn against lightning and the white lines around the barn door kept the devil out. Others believe these geometrical designs are symbols of witchcraft and hexerei to ward off evil spirits, fire, and sickness.

The hex sign came from the Cult of the Sun which was practiced during the Bronze Age. Since many residents of southeastern Pennsylvania came from Lower Saxony, Germany, at the beginning of the eighteenth century, these residents brought with them the geometric designs which they painted and carved on door frames and the wooden sides of the barns. Today, many of these geometric designs are being revived.

These geometric designs consisted of three basic figures: star, sunburst, and tear drop. The starlike designs were sun symbols. The sun was considered a source of light, heat, and life and also meant the source of goodness. The geometric designs were hex marks, witches' signs, or magic symbols to keep witches away from the family owning the barn. Hex designs had openings on the outside. The theory behind these openings was that the witch entered the opening, got tangled in the design, could not find her way out, and was trapped. The geometric designs had 4, 5, 6, 7, 8, 10, 12, 16, and 32 pointed stars. If an eight-pointed star was used, four colors were common: two shades of green, yellow, and a bright red center. A four-pointed star was referred as a good luck sign; a double eight-pointed star as a fertility sign; a four-pointed star with tear drops as a rain sign; and five-pointed star with a horse's head in the center as protection of livestock against disease. Also, the five-pointed star has been related to the five senses, protection against demons, and good luck. The circle has been associated with eternity.[9]

Powwowing is occult folk medicine that was brought to Eastern and Central Pennsylvania from the Rhineland of Germany and Switzerland in the eighteenth century. Although powwowing is forbidden by Protestant churches, powwowers treat persons with many diseases and chronic health conditions. Usually, the powwower does not mix one disease with another disease. The powwower must know the kind of pain to be treated. Powwowing is used because the ill person believes he is "hexed." To cure the "hexed" person, the powwower must "remove" the spell from the ill person and destroy the "witch" causing the hex by occult means. Thus, powwowing is "white magic." Present-day powwowers do not emphasize hexerei (witchcraft).

Rituals used by powwowers are developed by each powwower and involve chants in English or in Pennsylvania Dutch, charms, amulets, biblical verses, the trinitarian formula, Lord's Prayer, sign of the cross, and stroking the afflicted part of ill persons. Stroking is done in one direction and is a means of "collecting" the disease. In some cases the powwower may call upon powers of the supernatural world. Powwow charms are primitive and are set in a Christian frame with God the Father, God the Son, and God the Holy Ghost.

Powwowers operate on the fringe of the law. As long as the powwower does not charge a fee for the services or does not practice medicine, or the patient does not die because of the powwower's negligence, the powwower can practice powwowing.

Powwowers do not try to cure cancer or moles, but they have been known to treat corneal transplant, glaucoma, hemophilia, erysipelas, rheumatism, bleeding, inflammation, burns, warts, sinus, gallstones, asthma, infected glands of the neck, goiter, lumbago, bone abscess, arthritis, backache, gangrene and scurvy. Warts have been cured by cutting an onion in half, rubbing the halves on warts, putting the halves of onion together with a pin, burying the onion where rain water comes down, and repeating a Bible verse and the Lord's Prayer. A powwower treated a bone abscess by applying a black salve and stroking the abscess. Violent pains in the bones were treated by mixing prickly ash bark and rum and having the patient drink the concoction and rub the concoction over the pained area.[10]

CURANDERAS

In the Mexican-American culture, the curandera is a specialist in the diagnosis and treatment of illness based upon "folk theories and curing" of disease. These curanderas have more than the usual lay knowledge of Mexican folk medicine and may be paid a small fee for their services.

When a member of the family becomes ill, others in the family who have had experience with illness and "know about sickness and curing" are asked to diagnose and cure the ill person. If the illness cannot be diagnosed, the group calls upon friends and neighbors for suggestions.

Most frequently, the ill person sees a curandera before seeking proper medical care. One physician who has a large Mexican-American practice reported that at least 50 percent of all Spanish-speaking patients first consulted a curandera, regardless of the economic level of the patient.

The curanderas have no formal training in medicine and do not earn their living by curing. They are regarded as specialists because they have learned more of the popular folk medicine of their culture than other Mexican-Americans. Patients are often relatives, friends, and neighbors. Curanderas use the language of Spanish-speaking people, and their vocabularies consist of terms familiar to their patients.

When a curandera is asked to examine an ill person, the curandera is called upon both as a curer and a friend. The patient and members of the family know that the curandera is one of them and really cares about them. The patient is brought to the curandera's home. The patient and members of the family gather in the curandera's kitchen which smells of mint, rosemary, coriander, and cinnamon. The curandera is warm and friendly and observes the social amenities such as offering coffee and conversation to the family. The conversation is of weddings, social gatherings, and church bazaars—anything but the ill person. After a "decent" interval, the illness is mentioned and the patient is seen by the curandera.

Much information about the patient's illness has already been gathered by the curandera from neighborhood gossip. The curandera looks at the patient's eyes and color, feels the patient's pulse, and palpates the abdomen or calves of the legs. The diagnosis given by the curandera is one familiar to the patient and his family—*susto* or *bilis* or *mal ojo* or *mal aire*.

Treatment by the curandera may be started immediately, or instructions may be given to perform some treatment at home. If medication is prescribed, the curandera furnishes the ingredients from the curandera's herb garden or prescribes a simple and inexpensive medication that can be bought at a drugstore. Suggestions or criticisms for the treatment of the patient are always welcomed by the curandera. The family is free to accept or reject the treatment.

The curandera charges little or nothing for services to the patient. If the illness requires a medical doctor, the curandera recommends a physician who is *simpático* and inexpensive. Since most of the curandera's patients get well, the curandera has a devoted and grateful clientele. The curandera holds the confidence of families because the curandera fulfills the expectations of the curer as held by the Mexican-American culture.

Diseases are placed into these categories: diseases of dislocation of internal organs, diseases of "hot or cold" imbalance, diseases of magical origin, diseases of emotional origin, and "standard scientific" diseases.

Diseases of Dislocation of Internal Organs

An example of dislocation of internal organs is the *mollera caida* (fallen fontanelle) or the dropping of the anterior fontanelle of the infant's skull. One of the curandera's remedies for *mollera caida* is to hold the baby by the ankles, head down, and to dip the crown of the baby's head into hot water. Sometimes, the soles of the baby's feet are slapped while the baby is in the inverted position. Some curanderas recite prayers while the baby is in this position. Another remedy is the curandera's continuous pressure to the baby's hard palate with the fingertips. Or, the curandera places warm water in her mouth and sucks on the soft spot of the baby's skull. Or, the yolk of an egg is smeared on a piece of cigarette paper and pressed over the anterior fontanelle. Or, a thick paste of soap and table sugar is placed on the baby's fontanelle and removed after 24 hours.

Other diseases of dislocation of internal organs are growths or lumps in tissues of arms or legs and fallen uterus in women. The growths receive massage. The fallen uterus is "treated" by massage of the abdomen.

Diseases of Hot and Cold Imbalance

Burns are placed in this category. These diseases of "hot and cold" imbalance can be treated by "hot" and "cold" foods. Some hot foods are chili, garlic, crackles (pork rind), white beans, onions, pork, fish, capon, wheat bread, beans, potatoes, tortillas, honey, sugar, and salt. Among the cold foods are cucumbers, pickles, spinach, tomatoes, human milk, green beans, beets, cabbage, carrots, peas, pumpkin, radish, squash, beef, lamb, cow's milk, oatmeal, and turnips. Cold foods have been linked with head colds, colic, varicose veins, and death.

Hot and cold imbalance may be the reason for earache, head colds, pains in the joints, infant colic, tonsillitis or sore throat, nosebleeds, skin lesions and rashes, and backache. Nosebleed due to hot and cold imbalance is treated by two or three cold baths a day. Earache is treated by blowing hot air into the outer ear.

Women who are unable to conceive sit over a tub of hot water and rosemary. It is believed that the vapors from the water will warm the uterus and the woman can have a baby. Some of the hot substances used to aid conception are a plaster of belladonna leaves and a patent medicine, Brandreth's Pills. The plaster of belladonna leaves is placed over the sacral area each morning for several days. Brandreth's Pills consist of a cathartic, mandrake root, used for chronic constipation. The pills are taken with a cup of chocolate containing a little amount of powdered sulphur.

Diseases of Magical Origin

Diseases of magical origin are related to *mal ojo* or the "evil eye." Children and infants are the victims of *mal ojo*. A woman who admires someone else's child and looks at the child without touching the child may inflict the evil eye on the child. Some of the signs of the evil eye are continuous crying, diarrhea, fever, vomiting, and fitful sleep. The curandera diagnoses the evil eye by rubbing the child's body with a whole raw egg. The yolk of the egg is examined and if there is a red spot, the child has the evil eye.

The curandera treats mal ojo with eggs. An unbroken, fresh egg is held in the curandera's right hand and is used to make the sign of the cross on all parts of the child's body. The Apostles' Creed is recited three times. The egg is broken into a small bowl of water and six small pieces of palm are placed on the egg in the form of three small crosses. The child with *mal ojo* is put to bed and the bowl of water, egg, and palm are placed under his bed, directly below his head. The next morning if the egg looks cooked, the child is cured of *mal ojo*.

Evil spirits or other forces that are believed to inhabit the air, cause *mal aire* (bad air). The *mal aire* is the reason for different diseases and chronic health conditions. Epilepsy and dropsy are linked to *mal aire*.

Witchcraft or *brujeria* is regarded as a cause of many diseases, some of which may be malevolent. Prayers, religious objects such as pictures of saints, holy water, and spells are used to ward off evil forces. Infertility is often linked to witchcraft. One curandera treats barren women by suspending keys from the waist of the barren woman. The keys hang over the uterus and have been blessed. Often, a curandera will use herbs which she has blessed. Many people in the Mexican-American culture believe that *brujas* (witches) cause illness, but, none can describe the hexes or spells.

Diseases of Emotional Origin

Diseases of emotional origin are linked to emotional experiences producing fright, desire, embarrassment or shame, anger, disillusion, sadness, and imagined rejection. Anger *(bilis)* and fright *(susto)* are the two most common emotional experiences. The adult who becomes a victim of *bilis* first develops an uncontrollable rage and then a day or two later has acute nervous tension and chronic fatigue. Herbs are used to treat *bilis*. A tea made from boiling water, rosemary, camomile, and camphor leaf is drunk before breakfast on nine consecutive mornings. (*Three* and *nine* are thought to have a ritual significance.) Or, cassia bark, lemon shoots, whole lemon. cinnamon bark, and toasted walnut are added to a pint of whiskey. A half cup of this herbal concoction is taken before breakfast on nine consecutive mornings. Or, mint, fennel, dill, cassia bark, kernel of apricot seed, magnesium bicarbonate, peel of a sour orange, pomegranate seed, a few drops of lemon juice, and sugar are added to a small quantity of water and boiled in two cups of water. This herbal remedy is taken before breakfast for nine days.

Children who have experienced *susto* (fright) become pale and thin, have no appetite, have headaches, shake and tremble, and cannot stop being scared. The child being treated for *susto* must walk across a candle mounted in the middle of a saucer with a little water in it. After walking across the candle in one direction, the child crosses it again at right angles, making a cross. Then, branches of pepper leaves are swished from top to bottom and left to right, making a cross, over the child. The Apostles' Creed is recited. The child is put to bed under which are laid two pepper branches to form a cross. The curandera walks away from the bed, calling out: "Vente (child's name) no te quieres ni te espantes. (Come, _____ , you don't need anything and you aren't afraid.)" The cure is started before bedtime on a Wednesday night and is repeated on Thursday and Friday nights. After the third night, the child should be cured of *susto*.

Curanderas indicate that since *susto* is hard to cure a pregnant woman should avoid *susto* so that she will not give *susto* to the unborn child. If the pregnant woman has a bad fright, the woman drinks a glass of warm water with a few live coals and sugar to protect the baby from *susto*. Curanderas often claim that *el susto vieto* ("old fright") cannot be cured.

Standard Scientific Diseases

Standard scientific diseases known to the people of Mexican-American culture are measles, bronchitis, pneumonia, asthma, whooping cough, tuberculosis, sore throat, ulcer, cancer, appendicitis, head cold, and gallstones. A sore throat is believed to be caused by a foreign object such as a small red rat in the throat. Cancer is believed to be caused by eating artificial foods. Many phenomena such as loss of a lot of blood, a person perspiring and then drinking cold water, or a complication of a previous illness are accepted as the cause of tuberculosis. Often, diabetes is believed to be the cause of tuberculosis.

Patent medicines such as tonics, "cold medicine," cough syrups, laxatives, salves and liniments, alcohol, and vitamin preparations are used in treating standard scientific diseases. Vitamin pills may be taken for stomach trouble or postoperative care for cancer.[11]

FOLK MEDICINE

Due to the lack of medical doctors in remote areas of this country, folk medicine has become an acceptable way of life. Even in communities with modern medical research centers, folk medicine can thrive. Passed from generation to generation, folk medicine is a combination of fallacies about the use of herbs, poultices, and strange concoctions to cure diseases, remedy chronic health conditions, relieve miseries accompanying illness, and prevent other illnesses. Some examples are:

Pokeberry tea is a common drink of arthritis victims.
Teas made of boneset, whiskey and rock candy, and horehound are used to treat colds.
Red paper is given to persons with a sore throat.
Teas from hops and catnip are prepared for those with stomach trouble.
Fresh cow manure is made into a poultice to draw maggots out of sores.
Pulverized earth is placed over cuts.
Teas from sassafras are given to children each spring to thin, purify, and strengthen their blood.

Brown sugar is placed on a cut to stop the bleeding.
Bone is rubbed over a wart; then, the bone is buried where water dripped from eaves.
Asafetida is a preventative measure against diseases such as smallpox and whooping cough. It is taken internally for hysteria, diseases of females, colics and stomach trouble.

Asafetida, a member of the parsley family, is placed in a small bag and worn around the neck by children to prevent influenza. Or, bread and salt are added to the asafetida in the bag to keep evil spirits away and restore appetite. Bags were removed in the spring. Asafetida can be spelled *asafedity, assafedity,* or *asafetity.* At the beginning of the 20th century, asafetida, according to pharmocopeias, was a stimulant and antispasmodic for croup.

HEALTH FALLACIES

The number of health fallacies accepted by Americans has been a growing interest to many persons in the health professions, including the public health nurse, the family physician and dentist, pharmacist, hospital nurse, nutritionist, field workers of nonofficial health agencies, sanitarians, optometrist, physical therapist, podiatrist, social worker, and health educator. These fallacies result from beliefs passed from generation to generation, claims made by faddists, fear campaigns sponsored by groups opposing efforts to improve community health, biased propaganda distributed by cultists, and publications of quacks. Examples of these fallacies are quoted from *Focusing On Health.*[12]

Fallacies about the Care of the Human Body

"Deep breathing exercises increase the blood supply.
Regular strenuous exercise is harmful to the human heart.
A daily bath is necessary to prevent illness.
Everyone should take a laxative once a week.
A daily bowel movement is always necessary for good health.
Feet should form a forty-five degree angle if a person is to have good standing posture.
Sleeping on the left side of the body affects the heart.
Eye exercises prevent eye defects.
Sties are due to eating too much candy and reading too much.
Obesity is inherited.
Arch supports should be used by all people with flat feet.
It is a bad health habit to drink water while you exercise.
The best thing to do when your muscles are stiff is to work the stiffness out by taking vigorous exercise.
Regular exercise prevents diseases.
A pain in the lower back is a definite sign of kidney disease.
Bathing the eyes with cold water will improve vision.
A cold morning bath daily will make you immune to colds.
It is necessary for good health to keep the windows open in the bedroom at night.
Tobacco smoke is a good disinfectant.
Tobacco juice is a good antiseptic."

Fallacies about the Teeth

"Chewing gum prevents cavities.
The main purpose of toothpaste or tooth powder is to kill bacteria.
Mouthwashes kill all bacteria in the mouth and throat.

Care given to baby teeth is not important, since they are soon lost.
Bad breath is always a sign of poor health."

Fallacies about Diseases

"Boils are caused by bad blood in the human body.
Measles occurs only to children and pregnant women.
It is better for children to have such diseases as whooping cough, chicken pox, and scar-
let fever before they become twelve years of age.
Baking soda dissolved in water is a good cure for a cold.
Honey cures whooping cough.
Asafetida carried around the neck will ward off disease.
To cure a sore throat, wrap a wool sock around your throat.
Tonsillitis can be cured by hot pepper sauce.
Tuberculosis is inherited.
Tuberculin tests cause tuberculosis.
Overweight people never get tuberculosis.
A large chest and large lungs protect a person from tuberculosis.
Alcohol is a good remedy for colds.
Soaking the feet in hot water will cure a cold.
Vaccinations against polio, smallpox, and tetanus do not prevent these diseases.
Sickness is a punishment for being bad.
A child with rheumatic fever will never fully recover.
The best medicines are the medicines that taste the worst.
Watermelons and cucumbers cause polio."

Fallacies about Chronic Health Conditions

"Cancer is contagious.
Cancer is not curable.
All types of cancer are inherited.
Diabetes is caused by eating too many sweet foods.
Huckleberry tea will cure diabetes.
Olive oil will prevent appendicitis.
Blueberry juice will rid the body of diabetes.
Diabetes is the result of an injury to the liver.
All epileptics are mentally retarded.
Cases of glaucoma always result in blindness.
Drinking ice water causes heart disease.
To get rid of a cataract in the eye grind up eggshells into a powder and sprinkle into
the eye.
There is no education or help for persons with cerebral palsy.
Total deafness is the result of overhearing conversations not meant to be heard.
Muscular dystrophy strikes after injuries to muscles.
Arthritis can be cured.
An arthritic cannot eat meat or drink milk."

Fallacies about Menstruation

"Certain foods cannot be eaten during menstruation.
It's risky to shampoo the hair when menstruating.
Menstrual blood is bad blood.
If a dentist puts in a filling during the girl's menstrual period, the filling won't stay in.
Taking a bath during menstruation will cause tuberculosis.
Eating a lemon will start the menstrual period ahead of time.
A girl menstruating cannot take care of a younger brother because she will make him
sick.
Loss of menstrual blood weakens the girl.
People always know when a girl is menstruating.
A girl who is menstruating should not touch milk, since she will cause the milk to
curdle."

Fallacies about Fluoridation of Drinking Water

"Fluoridated water is poisonous.
Fluoridation is a communist plot.
Children are born defective because their mother drank fluoridated water.
Cancer is caused by fluoridation.
Fluoridation damages internal organs of the human body.
Acne is aggravated by fluoridation.
Fluoridation makes the bones brittle.
The physical development of children is retarded by fluoridation.
Fluoridation causes the hair to fall out."

Fallacies about Warts, Earache, Painful Corn, Insanity, and Freckles

"To get rid of moles and warts, tie a string around them.
If you handle a toad, you will get warts on your hands.
A wart can be removed by rubbing a key over it.
Blow smoke into the ear to cure an earache.
If your corn hurts, it is a reliable sign that it is going to rain.
A person will become insane if the moon shines upon his face while he is sleeping.
Buttermilk will remove freckles.
Man has one less rib than woman."

Fallacies about Carbohydrates

"Toast has fewer calories than bread.
A gelatin dessert is nonfattening.
Enriched bread has fewer vitamins than home-baked bread.
Bananas make people overweight.
Home-ground flour is more nutritious than commercially ground flour.
Rice cures high blood pressure.
Dry cereals supply all needed body energy.
Blackstrap molasses cures arthritis.
Gelatin strengthens the fingernails."
Dark bread has fewer calories than white bread per slice.
Millers remove from bread twenty nutrients and add only four nutrients.

Fallacies about Fats

"Margarine has fewer calories than butter.
Margarine is hard to digest.
Fat meat gives people strength.
Water turns to fat within the body.
Frozen desserts made with vegetable fat have no calories.
Meat is fattening.
Butter should not be eaten after taking penicillin.
Margarine adversely affects the depth of the voice."
Popcorn is a good meat substitute.
Eating meat in usual amounts damages the liver and kidneys.

Fallacies about Proteins

"Fish and celery are brain foods.
White eggs are more nutritious than brown eggs.
Raw eggs are more nutritious than cooked eggs.
Beef liver is more nutritious than pork liver.
Rare beefsteaks provide more energy than steaks that are well-done.
Cheese is hard to digest.
A person with arthritis should not eat meat and eggs.
Proteins and starches should not be eaten at the same meal.
A well-conditioned athlete has need for more protein than a less active person."

Fallacies about Vitamins

"Taking vitamin pills will ensure good health.
Vitamin pills can cure most diseases.
If one vitamin pill a day is good, two or three vitamin pills are better.
Vitamins need not be prescribed by physicians.
Vitamin C (ascorbic acid) is stored in the body.
Potatoes have no vitamins.
Vitamins provide the human body with sufficient calories.
Vitamins rebuild blood.
Vitamins take the place of iron in the human body."

Fallacies about Milk

"Thunder causes milk to sour.
Raw milk is the best quality milk.
Milk is constipating.
Milk is hard to digest.
Milk is for children, not for adults.
Milk should not be given to a person with a fever.
Sour cream has fewer calories than sweet cream.
Yogurt provides more nutrients than whole milk.
Homogenized milk contains no fat.
Milk combined with chili, lettuce, fish, lemons, tomatoes, cherries, cucumbers, spinach, oysters, or cabbage causes illness."
Cold milk is harmful to most children.

Fallacies about Beverages

"Wine makes blood.
Port wine is good for the liver.
Uncolored carbonated drinks have no calories.
Sassafras tea thins the blood.
Rheumatism can be cured by alfalfa tea.
Grape juice cures cancer.
Coffee is a depressant to the central nervous system."
Coffee increases efficiency in learning.
"Beer has no calories.
Alcoholic beverages contain all needed nutrients."
Desire for alcoholic beverages is passed from parent to child.

Fallacies about Fruits and Vegetables

"Tomatoes are a tonic for the liver.
Celery cures rheumatism.
Beets cleanse the blood.
If an orange is eaten every day, a person's blood will dry up.
Swallowing the seeds of grapes causes appendicitis.
Ripe cherries restore worn-out body tissues.
All fruits and vegetables should be eaten raw.
Frozen orange juice is less nutritious than fresh orange juice.
Canned vegetables are always less nutritious than fresh, cooked vegetables.
Vegetable juices are more nutritious than fresh vegetables."
Asparagus cures diseases of the kidneys.
Apple cider vinegar and lemon juice enable the person to burn fat instead of storing it.
Sour fruits like lemons cause acid stomach or heartburn.

Fallacies about Weight Reduction

"Skipping meals is a good way to lose weight.
If you take reducing pills, you can eat all you want.

Washing rice after cooking reduces the number of calories.
When trying to lose weight, a person should not drink water.
High protein foods have no calories.
Grapefruit will cause a person to lose weight.
Fruit has no calories.
Sugar is not as fattening as starch.
Omitting breakfast is a good way to lose weight.
Candy enriched with vitamins will hasten weight loss.
Tomatoes or pineapple with a meal brings about reduction in weight."
Most persons are overweight because of the fattening foods they eat rather than the amount of food they eat.

Miscellaneous Fallacies about Nutrition

"Additional food is needed for mental activity.
Green glass jars keep all foods from spoiling.
Cooking foods in aluminum utensils will cause cancer.
Give a child all the food he wants, and he will never suffer from malnutrition.
You should starve a fever and feed a cold.
If you are hungry all the time, you have a tapeworm.
It is dangerous to eat when taking sulfa drugs.
Eating at irregular hours causes stomach trouble."
A person's health status is not affected by what he eats.
A good way to digest food is to smoke a cigarette after eating.

Fallacies promoted by food faddists such as soil depletion, chemical fertilizers poisoning the land, foods having magical powers, and subclinical deficiencies were presented in Chapter 2. Fallacies used by quacks, such as cancer quacks, were given in Chapter 1.

REFERENCES

1. Douglas, M. (editor): Witchcraft: Conferences and Accusations. London, Tavistock Publications, 1970. Holzer, H.: The Truth About Witchcraft. Garden City, New York, Doubleday & Company, Inc., 1969. Tindall, G.: A Handbook on Witches. London, Arthur Barker Limited, 1965.
2. Huebner, L.: Power Through Witchcraft. Los Angeles, Nash Publishing Corp., 1969, p. 9.
3. Huxley, F.: The Invisibles. London, Rupert Hart-Davis, 1966, pp. 85, 239.
4. Webb, J. Y.: Superstitious Influence—Voodoo in Particular—Affecting Health Practices in a Selected Population in Southern Louisiana. New Orleans, published by the author, 1971, pp. 8-96.
5. Gibbs, S.: Voodoo practices in modern New Orleans. Louisiana Folklore Miscellany, 3:12 1971.
6. McTeer, J. E.: High Sheriff of the Low Country. Beaufort, South Carolina, Beaufort Book Company, Inc., 1970, pp. 19-42.
7. Michaelson, M.: Can a "Root Doctor" actually put a hex on or is it all a great put on? Today's Health, 50:39, 1972.
8. McTeer, op. cit.
9. Smith, E. L.: Hex Signs and Other Barn Decorations. Lebanon, Pennsylvania, Applied Arts Publishers, 1965, pp. 4-5, 6, 8-9.
10. Snellenburg, B.: Four Interviews with powwowers. Pennsylvania Folklife, 28:40, 1969. Westkott, M.: Powwowing in Berks County. Pennsylvania Folklife, 29:2, 1970. Yoder, D.: Twenty questions on powwowing. Pennsylvania Folklife, 15:38, 1966.
11. Clark, M.: Health in the Mexican American Culture. Los Angeles, University of California Press, 1970, pp. 162-211.
12. Haag, J.: Focusing On Health. Austin, Texas, Steck-Vaughn Company, 1973, pp. 17-24.

SUPPLEMENTAL READINGS

Huson, P.: Mastering Witchcraft: A Practical Guide for Witches, Warlocks, and Covens. New York, G. P. Putnam's Sons, 1970.

Leek, S.: Diary of a Witch. Englewood Cliffs, New Jersey, Prentice-Hall, Inc., 1968.

Mair, L. P.: Witchcraft. New York, McGraw-Hill Book Company, 1969.

Martinez, R.: Mysterious Marie Laveau—Voodoo Queen. New Orleans, Hope Publications, 1956.

Middleton, J.: Magic, Witchcraft, and Curing. New York, American Museum of Natural History, 1967.

Pelton, R. W.: The Complete Book of Voodoo. New York, G. P. Putnam's Sons 1972.

Rigaud, M.: Secrets of Voodoo. New York, Arco Company, 1969.

Smith, S.: Today's Witches. Englewood Cliffs, New Jersey, Prentice-Hall, Inc., 1970.

Tallant, R.: Voodoo in New Orleans. New York, Collier Books, 1962.

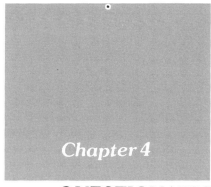

Chapter 4

QUESTIONABLE HEALTH CARE

WITH the increases in hospital and physicians' fees, many adults are seeking other sources of health care. This chapter raises questions about health care given by nursing homes, clinics, health care imposters, unethical doctors, naturopaths, chiropractors, and unqualified physicians.

NURSING HOMES

Four major types of nursing homes meeting different medical needs exist in the United States. The *extended-care facility* (ECF) usually operates in connection with a hospital and offers around-the-clock nursing services and medical supervision. ECF's patients are cases of medical necessity. For patients 65 years of age or older, Medicare will pay a portion of the cost of care in nursing homes after the hospital stay. Many private health insurance policies also pay for stays in extended-care facilities. A skilled-nursing home has patients who are not well enough to stay home or do not need the intensive care of ECF's. Trained nurses are supposed to be on hand at all times. Medicare will pay the bills if a physician orders a patient 65 years of age or older into such a facility. The *intermediate care facility,* called a nursing home by most people, is for those patients who need help with problems of their daily lives and continuous care of their general health. A *residential home* offers no medical or nursing care and is not supervised by governmental agencies.

More than one million Americans are in nursing homes. Their average age is 82 years; 3 of every 4 patients are women; and 92 percent are white. The patients are afflicted with these disabilities: cardiovascular diseases, fractures, arthritis, and senility. Their average length of stay in a nursing home is 2 or more years.

Considered to be one of the fastest growing industries, nursing homes collected more than $8 billion in 1974. Before Medicaid and in 1960, public payments for nursing home care amounted to $500 million. In 1974, $4 billion went to nursing homes from Medicaid. There were fewer than 10,000 nursing homes and 331,000 beds in 1960. At least 23,000 nursing homes with 1.2 million beds existed in 1974.

Good nursing homes, meeting state and federal regulations, are found throughout the United States. Inflation, rising labor costs, and tight money have closed some small nursing homes and resulted in expanding waiting lists for those able to operate. Many items such as medicine, food, and fuel have risen in cost more than the cost-of-living index. Employees have become unionized and pushed up labor costs. Tightness of money for construction has limited the building or expansion of nursing homes.

The rapid expansion of the nursing home industry and funds from Medicare and Medicaid have resulted in a proliferation of unlicensed facilities and other nursing homes failing to meet standards of acceptability. Congress, state and local agencies, and the Department of Health, Education, and Welfare are investigating charges of neglect to patients, fraud, and unsanitary facilities in nursing homes.

Other charges of kickbacks, padding of payrolls, and fire hazards are being cited by state authorities. The Department of Health, Education, and Welfare is not the only federal agency interested in the nursing home industry. The Internal Revenue Service and the Securities and Exchange Commission have started investigating nursing homes with corporate status.

Investigation of charges has revealed cruelty to patients, neglect of patients, unsanitary food handling, virulent infections among patients, unsanitary facilities, callousness on the part of nursing home administrators and employees, and unnecessary regimentation of patients. Patients who urinate or have a bowel movement without any knowledge that these bodily functions have occurred may not receive any attention for several hours. There may be no privacy for the patient, no call bell handy, no bed permitting the ambulatory patient to get in and out of bed easily, and no clean toilet and bathing facilities. There may be no physical therapy, no recreational facilities, and no special diet for the patient. The visiting hours may be restricted so that friends and relatives cannot visit as easily as they should. Virulent infections such as common colds, streptococcal sore throat, staphylococcal infections, and influenza may be spread from one patient to the next patient. Patients have died from beatings and other maltreatment.

Not all family physicians continue their supervision when their patients are placed in nursing homes. Family physicians may assume that owners of nursing homes who are physicians will assume personal attention of their former patients. Too often, the owner-physician has no contact with nursing home patients unless a patient dies or there is an emergency.

Few of the nation's registered professional nurses work in nursing homes. Those professional nurses in nursing homes devote most of their time to administrative duties. Eighty to 90 percent of nursing-home care is provided by licensed vocational or practical nurses, nurse's aides, and orderlies. Too often, care is given by persons who have no preparation for the job. With no understanding of rheumatoid arthritis or osteoarthritis, the so-called nurse can cruelly injure the arthritic by forcing movement in an arthritic hand, knee, or foot. Often these ill-trained "nurses" give their version of physical therapy or ignore the physical exercises needed by the patient. Many persons providing nursing-home care become calloused in their treatment of elderly or incurably ill patients.

Danger of fires in nursing homes is commonly reported in investigations. At least 72 percent of nursing homes have one or more violations of building codes. Poor construction of buildings, faulty electrical connections, poorly operated heating and ventilation systems, inadequate trash disposal methods, fire hazards in the kitchen and garage, flammable interior decorations and furniture, and inadequate numbers of fire escapes and doors are some of the causes of nursing home tragedies. In 1974, there were 4800 nursing-home fires, and more than 500 persons were killed.

From 20 to 40 percent of drugs given to patients in nursing homes are in error. The nursing-home patient's bill for drugs is more than triple that of noninstitutionalized elderly persons. Kickbacks to owners of nursing homes by pharmacists are widespread. Many over-the-counter and prescription drugs are given to nursing home patients who do not need the drugs, and tranquilizers are often administered to keep patients docile. Drug prescriptions may be renewed without a physician's approval and supervision.

In addition to the deficiencies of nursing homes, forthright standards to provide patients with minimum protection are not enforced. Standards are so vague that state and local agencies cannot enforce them even though some agencies do a good job. Improvement in long-term care for older Americans is one of the reforms most needed in the health-care system.

CLINICS

"Fat clinics" are widely advertised between Chicago and the West Coast. These weight-reduction clinics provide human chorionic gonadotropin (HCG) injections under directions of physicians. Large sums of money are offered to physicians to affiliate with these clinics. Most medical experts agree that HCG, made from urine of pregnant women, does not reduce obesity. The HCG clinics place their patrons on 500-calorie-a-day diets.[1]

The Contreras Clinic, Tijuana, Mexico, treats cancer victims by offering Laetrile. Many of the cancer victims are Americans who travel across the border to receive Laetrile which cannot be prescribed in the United States. At the clinic the victims are told to stop the medication prescribed by American physicians and to take two or three pills of Laetrile each day for complete cancer cures. While at the Clinic, the patient pays $15 cash for three daily injections. Laetrile, which is derived from apricot kernels, is believed to break down into several components when inside the human body. One of these components is said to be a cyanide poison that chokes off the cancerous tumor. Autopsies have shown consistent progression of cancer, even though the persons had made several trips to the Contreras Clinic.[2]

There are 3500 to 5000 "sex clinics" or "sex treatment centers" in the United States. Possibly no more than 50 offer treatment methods with proper scientific care, have undergone conscientious testing and evaluation, and are administered by trained and competent personnel. Undercover investigations of phony sex clinics have revealed self-styled therapists who were criminals, mentally ill, or unqualified practitioners. Some phony clinics advertise or privately assure patients that their therapists are "Masters-and-Johnson-trained therapists" or that their treatment is based on "the M-J technique." These claims are not true. Some phony sex clinics have therapists who seduce clients either homosexually or heterosexually and charge exorbitant fees. Once the person has undergone quack sex therapy, it is increasingly difficult for the person to seek legitimate sex counseling and psychotherapy.[3]

Rejuvenation was offered by the "New Life Clinic," Fort Myers, Florida.[4] The Clinic provided cellular therapy to patients who paid $1000 apiece for a set of 10 injections into the buttocks within a 7-minute period. The injections were live cells from the organs of the fetus of a sheep, which were supposed to reverse the aging process of specific human organs. Heart cells of the fetus, for example, would purportedly reverse the aging process of the patients' heart cells. After two deaths from gas gangrene, the Florida Board of Osteopathic Medicine and the Florida State Attorney filed formal charges against the owner.[4]

HEALTH CARE IMPOSTERS

Medical imposters are persons who desire the respect and status of licensed physicians, whose lives have been failures, and who are fascinated by the spell of medicine. One of them was a laboratory technician who applied for a position as a physician in a hospital. His qualifications included graduation from medical school, internship, medical practice in a large city, and instructor in hematology in a prestigious university. When the hospital checked with the American Medical Association's Department of Investigation, the qualifications were nonexistent.

Some imposters assume the name of a licensed physician. "Doctor" Reed L. Brown established his practice when he stopped for a soda at a drugstore in a small Texas town that had lost its only medical doctor. A child with a severe gash in his leg was brought in, and "Dr." Brown volunteered to stitch the gash. He soon had a busy practice, but was forced to relinquish it after a computer of a drug manufacturer detected that two physicians of the same name and credentials were prescribing drugs. Brown had "lifted" the name and credentials of a licensed physician.

Another imposter obtained reading lists of premedical courses, bought and read the books of the courses, and visited courses at Johns Hopkins in Baltimore and Wayne State University Medical School in Detroit in addition to spending time in hospitals associated with these medical schools. He prepared a phony diploma and hung out a shingle. When he applied for a life insurance policy, his impersonation was discovered.

Ferdinand W. Demara has impersonated a Catholic priest, a penologist, the dean of the school of philosophy in a college, a teacher of French and Latin, and a surgeon-lieutenant in the Royal Canadian Navy. Demara acquired the credentials of Joseph C. Cyr, a licensed Canadian physician. As Lieutenant Joseph C. Cyr, Demara was placed on duty at a naval hospital where he studied a medical guide prepared by the senior medical officer and watched other physicians in surgery and in patients' rooms. Assigned to duty on a Canadian aircraft carrier he suppressed a report about his inadequate preparation in medical diagnosis and surgery and circumvented any action against himself by hiding patients about whose conditions he felt unsure. These patients were placed in a quarantine area and given penicillin. Later, as the ship's doctor on a Canadian destroyer, this medical imposter did emergency surgery on 19 badly wounded men found at sea. When Navy dispatches carried the account of the emergency surgery, the story was reported by Canadian newspapers. The real Dr. Joseph C. Cyr asked authorities some probing questions, and the hoax was discovered.[5]

UNETHICAL DOCTORS

Luis Carrillo, M.D., Mexicali, Mexico, has convinced his patients that he can reduce the pain of arthritis and cure the arthritis victim. The Mexican Rheumatism Society has reported that Dr. Carrillo has "not found the cure for anything" and that the Society cannot recommend him.[6] Although patients of Dr. Carrillo have stated that the doctor has studied and taught at the Mayo Clinic, the Mayo Clinic has issued a public statement that it has no affiliation with Dr. Carrillo.

Artruro Diaz Montes, M.D., Dr. Carrillo's uncle, treats arthritic patients with corticosteroids. Both are reported to prescribe drugs in an indiscriminate manner. Dr. Carrillo hands the patient prescription slips to be taken to a designated pharmacy. The drugs may cost several hundreds of dollars, since the medication is to last for several months or until the next trip to Dr. Carrillo. Often the drugs prescribed could be dangerous. By ethical standards of medicine, Drs. Carrillo and Montes "misrepresent what they do prescribe and compound their wrong doing by providing little or no supervision and follow-up."[6]

Both Dr. Carrillo and Dr. Montes examine patients hurriedly and incompletely. Dr. Carrillo "sees" at least 120 patients in a 10-hour working day. The average examination lasts no more than 7 minutes. Many of the patients are 60 years of age and older, and their illnesses are usually not properly diagnosed.

Samuel Cole Fulkerson joined with John A. Restifo, sometimes claiming to be an M.D. and sometimes to have a Ph.D. in chemistry, to found the National Scientific Laboratories for treatment of the *healthy*. A client, with or without a physician's recommendation, would send a urine sample and receive a dire-sounding report, e.g., "impaired body chemistry." The urinalysis report would be analyzed by Nutritional Research Associates (Fulkerson and an associate, Carl R. Nelson, D.O.) who would prescribe appropriate vitamins from Professional Foods (Fulkerson and salesmen in the field).

A specimen of "urine" sent to Nelson and Fulkerson was some imitation urine made from demineralized distilled water, vegetable coloring, a drop of Lugol's iodine solution, and a dash of urea. By the time Nelson and Fulkerson had "analyzed" it, they had discovered androgens, ketosteroids, and corticoids in "low normal range." When other batches of synthetic urine were sent to Nelson and Fulkerson, the "analyses" showed numerous different hormones. With that and other information, the Postal Inspection Service indicted Fulkerson and Nelson who were convicted of mail fraud. During the time Fulkerson, Restifo, and Nelson had operated their fraudulent schemes, $3 million had been spent on urinalyses and $8 million on vitamins.[7]

Psychic surgeons claim to "operate" on patients by plucking out offending tumors, piercing the patient's skin with their bare hands, and painlessly removing circulatory blocks or other abnormalities without anesthetia or surgical instruments. The time of the average operation is 15 to 20 minutes. One of the most renowned psychic surgeons is Anthony Agpaoa, or Dr. Tony or Rev. Tony, of Manila, who has collected "donations" in excess of $1 million from more than 1000 persons from the state of Washington.

Twenty "tourists" or prospective clients will travel from a West Coast airport to Manila, where they are housed in the downtown hotel in which the psychic surgeons have a two-room suite. In the "operating room" the patient is told to lie on a table. A sheet is draped over the area of the body where the patient's medical doctor has located a malignant tumor. Dr. Tony rubs his salves into that area and then covers it with a six-inch square of cotton soaked with a liquid. Next, blood splatters the sheet, and Dr. Tony holds up a gory strip of fleshy tissue, which an aide snips free. An assistant wipes the "operated" site clean of blood, and the diseased area is "whole" again.

Actually, no incision was made and no tissue was removed, but there were sleight-of-hand tricks. A strip of animal flesh and capsules of animal blood or other red liquids were either "palmed" or hidden in the cotton, or the cotton had been soaked in a clear, water-like substance that turned blood red when a baking soda solution was added.[8]

ACUPUNCTURE

American medicine has initiated vigorous investigations concerning the use of acupuncture for anesthesia and the treatment of deafness, narcotics withdrawal, and chronic pain. Many of the acupuncture clinics in the United States are not affiliated with medical schools or major hospitals. Some do not have a licensed medical doctor to supervise the treatment. Often the clinics have "acupuncturists" with dubious or non-existent training and credentials. In the United States, probably no more than a "few dozen" practitioners of acupuncture have been adequately trained. Many are unqualified nonmedical people who "moonlight" as acupuncturists. Some "clinics" claim that their acupuncturists have trained for more than 10 years or that their patients have "good results" after a few treatments. Other clinics give glittering promises of relief from pain, arthritis, headaches, neuralgia, and joint pains.[9]

Quacks are sometimes found in acupuncture clinics for nerve deafness. One clinic advertised that its patients "responded well" to acupuncture treatment for nerve deafness. Another clinic claimed that patients began to hear better after a few treatments. Still another clinic sent a letter to prospective patients stating that its staff of medical doctors and acupuncturists had developed techniques that improved hearing.[9] Even though some patients have had partial hearing restored in acupuncture clinics, most medical doctors and scientists using acupuncture have been cautious in their conclusions about the benefits of acupuncture in the treatment of deafness.

Needles are inserted into the patient's inner ear in the use of acupuncture to reduce the pains of withdrawal from heroin. After the addict has received acupuncture treatments for a number of weeks with three half-hour sessions each day, he may notice reduction in aching, nausea, cramps, and runny eyes and nose. As the pains of withdrawal are reduced, the former addict participates in an overall rehabilitation program and methadone maintenance. Insufficient data have not shown that acupuncture is more effective than methadone maintenance alone with former heroin addicts.

Relief of chronic pain is the major goal of many persons who have neuralgia, migraine headaches, osteoarthritis, low back pain, sciatica, and joint pains. Reduction of pain through acupuncture treatments appears to be unpredictable. Some patients experience long-term remission of pain, but others receive only temporary relief.

The most promising application of acupuncture is as surgical anesthesia for root canal therapy in dentistry, skin grafts, tumor biopsies, tonsillectomies, and appendectomies. However, the medical profession in the United States does not accept acupuncture for this purpose.

Many states insist that acupuncture be done by a licensed physician and have strict licensing requirements for the professional acupuncturists. Those licensed physicians who do acupuncture perform it under the auspices of a hospital or a medical school.[10]

NATUROPATHS

If licensed, naturopaths are confined by statute to the use of natural remedies. Naturopaths do *not* use roentgenograms, prescribe drugs (except those drugs occurring naturally), or perform surgery. There are no specific naturopathic hospitals in the United States, and naturopaths do not have hospital privileges.[11]

Naturopathic medicine has been defined as the "prevention and treatment of disease by using biochemical, psychological, and physical methods that assist the resident healing processes of the body."[12] Naturopathic medicine is based upon the philosophy that man is subject to natural laws in health and disease. These laws include physiological, mental, and mechanical principles of life, which establish a balance within the human body. When this balance is upset, ill health and disease result. Any treatment that violates these laws is considered unnatural.

The four fields of naturopathic medicine are:
1. Body mechanics: anatomical manipulations, remedial exercises, and prosthetics.
2. Corrective nutrition: dietetics, food supplements, vitamins, minerals, botanicals, and other natural preparations.
3. Physiotherapy: natural physical agents including water, light, heat, electricity, and ultrasound.
4. Remedial psychology: psychosomatics and therapy.

Courses of study include basic sciences, clinical diagnosis, radiology, physical medicine, remedial psychology, naturopathic medicine, body mechanics, corrective nutrition, and biochemistry.[13] Naturopaths may claim that they are capable of treating any health condition seen in routine medical practice.

At the ninety-seventh annual meeting of the American Public Health Association, this resolution concerning naturopaths and chiropractors was adopted:

"3. That state legislatures and health agencies not include chiropractors and naturopaths under state health programs.
4. That states reevaluate their existing licensure programs for chiropractors and natur-

paths to determine whether such licenses should be further restricted or abolished, and that existing restrictions be more vigorously policed.

5. That professional and consumer groups undertake appropriate consumer education on the hazards of unscientific health care including chiropractic and naturopathy."[14]

CHIROPRACTORS

Derived from two Greek words meaning "done by hands," chiropractic is based upon the belief that diseases, chronic health conditions such as diabetes, and many other physical and mental illnesses are caused by subluxations of the vertebrae that can be diagnosed by spinal analyses and treated by manipulations of the spine or "chiropractic adjustment." A subluxation is a misalignment of vertebrae that pinches the nerves leaving the spinal cord. This pinching reduces the flow of "nerve force" to an organ of the human body.[15] The *Bulletin of the Palmer College of Chiropractic* describes chiropractic as follows:

"A subluxated vertebra, interfering with the normal nerve supply of an organ, brings about functional disease which may be followed by pathological disease.

"The chiropractor, having established a disease has been caused by subluxated vertebra, directs his efforts to determining which vertebra is subluxated, and to the adjustment of this vertebra back to its normal range of movement. Following the adjustment, the normal nerve supply is restored to the organ or system of organs, and their normal function may be reestablished.

"Chiropractors, through careful analysis of the entire spine, may not only locate the subluxated vertebra, but through nerve fiber distribution may locate the region of the affected organ. They may then advise the patient about the nature of his symptoms, and suggest methods of care for the body while it is being restored to a normal state of health."[16]

Chiropractic Treatment

A report by the Department of Health, Education, and Welfare in 1968 stated that chiropractors "treat nearly every type of illness."[17] A survey by the American Chiropractic Association revealed that 81 percent of the chiropractors "indicated that conditions other than musculoskeletal ranked first, second, or third among conditions most frequently treated."[18] From the survey, chiropractors stated that they treated the following conditions: "headache, 98 percent; asthma, 76 percent; chronic heart condition, 70 percent; mental, emotional, 68 percent; polio, 47 percent; pneumonia, 32 percent; appendicitis, 30 percent; leukemia, 8 percent; and cancer, 7 percent."[19]

When a patient visits the chiropractor for the first time, a spinal analysis is made by the chiropractor running his fingers slowly and evenly down the vertebrae. The subluxation or subluxations are named. This is the cause of the patient's disease, chronic health condition such as asthma, mental illness, pain, or other physical discomfort. The chiropractor explains that subluxations "'cause the nerve impulses to go either too fast or too slow' causing the organs served by these haywire nerves to function incorrectly."[20]

Two 36 x 14 inch "full spine" radiograms are usually made, one from the front and one from the side. These spinograph films are used for diagnosis of patients with "appendicitis, asthma, back injury, constipation, diabetes, irregular menses, nervous breakdown, 'disabled by pain,' prostate disorder, sciata, sciatic rheumatism, migrane headaches, heart condition, ear and throat abscesses, pain in kidneys, and lumbago and sciatica."[21] Spinographs may be made by the chiropractor once a month, every three months, or every six months.

The treatment consists mainly of spinal adjustments with heavy downward thrusts on the patient's spinal vertebrae by the chiropractor. The pressure can include all of the chiropractor's weight and strength. In addition to the thrusts, the head and neck may be jerked violently.[22] The average number of adjustments reported by chiropractors for 250,000 cases is given in Table 4-1.[23]

TABLE 4-1
CHIROPRACTIC ADJUSTMENTS FOR VARIOUS DISORDERS[23]

Condition	Average Number of Adjustments
Acne	28.2
Angina pectoris	32.1
Appendicitis	22.3
Arthritis	49.0
Deafness	33.2
Diabetes	51.3
Epilepsy	76.1
Eye disorders	42.5
Goiter	43.3
Heart disorders	36.8
Hemorrhoids	50.9
High blood pressure	32.1
Jaundice	84.1
Kidney disorders	43.2
Menstrual disorders	33.1
Nephritis	34.1
Obesity	47.3
Palsy	63.7
Parkinson's disease	57.6
Pneumonia	28.6
Polio (acute)	34.6
Polio (chronic)	51.3
Prostate trouble	42.9
Rheumatic fever	52.2
Ulcers	46.2

Chiropractors have used many types of mechanical gadgets, some of which have later been banned by the Food and Drug Administration. One of the early devices for diagnosis was the Neurocalometer which supposedly indicated warm spots where subluxations were located. Another diagnostic device was the Micro-Dynameter which had two electrodes of different metals and a quivering needle on a dial. Accompanying the Micro-Dynameter was a chart which correlated the readings on the dial with vitamins the patient should receive. If the Micro-Dynameter indicated that the sixth dorsal vertabra was subluxated, then vitamin No. 6 was recommended. When Food and Drug Administration officials applied the Micro-Dynameter to two cadavers, the machine indicated the cadavers were in perfect health.

The Detoxacolon was an example of a device sold by mail by a chiropractor for treatment of cancer, epilepsy, asthma, high and low blood pressure, and arthritis. Patients who responded to the advertisement for a free medical examination by a "famous diagnostician" would be told they needed a series of Detoxacolon treatments consisting of irrigations of the colon with water and oxygen.

Some of the mechanical devices used for diagnosis and treatment in the Drown Laboratories operated by two chiropractors were described in Chapter 1. A chiropractor used one of the Drown therapy devices on a client who had polyps in the lower intestines. The Drown gadget showed no cancer, even though the client's condition became worse while the Drown gadget was being used. The client died of cancer. It was claimed that the Drown gadgets could cure every known affliction, including those not discovered by medical science.[24]

Professional Training

Chiropractors earn their degrees in colleges of chiropractic rather than in medical schools. Today there are ten colleges of chiropractic. A survey of the courses listed in the catalogs of these colleges reveals that the curricula apparently include many of the courses that might be found in curricula for allied health, natural sciences, undergraduate medicine, and medical specialties.[25-34] Frequently the courses are classified as basic sciences and clinical sciences as they might be in a medical school catalog. In addition, there are courses in chiropractic philosophy, principles, techniques, clinic, spinography, office procedures, and X-ray.

Critics have maintained, however, that chiropractors are not trained for comprehensive medical care, and for a number of years chiropractic was not included under Medicare. The American Medical Association has stated that chiropractic is "an unscientific cult whose practitioners lack the necessary training and background to diagnose and treat human illnesses.[35] The questions about the legitimacy of chiropractic may be resolved by a study to be conducted by the National Institute of Neurological Diseases and Stroke.

The College of Physicians and Surgeons of the Province of Quebec submitted, in 1963, to the Royal Commission on Chiropractic the following statements:

> "Chiropractors claim that subluxations, or partial displacements of the vertebrae cause a perturbation of the distribution of nervous impulses to tissues and cells. Neurophysiologists have developed methods of recording the passage of impulses in nerves. Exceptionally sensitive apparatus is available to anyone wishing to use it. No scientific study has been published on the subject by a chiropractor. No chiropractor has ever defined, either quantitatively or qualitatively, what chiropractic means by perturbation of nervous impulses. Is it their number, their amplitude, their frequency, the speed of their propagation, or their wave patterns which are affected? All of these qualities can be identified, recorded, and studied. . . . Chiropractors affirm that alterations in the distribution of nervous impulses to tissues and cells disturb the state of health and provoke the illnesses which they treat. By what experimental proof have they demonstrated a causative relationship between disturbances of nervous flow and the development of the illnesses they claim to cure? Here again, absolutely none."[36]

In 1968, the Department of Health, Education, and Welfare presented to the United States Congress an exhaustive study of chiropractors as unacceptable practitioners in the Medicare program. The HEW report, in evaluating chiropractic education, not only found lack of qualified faculty but also extremely low admission requirements, high student-faculty ratios, inadequate facilities and libraries, lack of inpatient hospital experience, and no reports of adequate basic scientific research by the faculties. "These shortcomings raise serious doubts as to the qualifications of chiropractors generally to make an adequate diagnosis and effectively treat patients," the report stated. "The doubts are compounded when seen in light of chiropractic philosophy."[37]

The 1968 HEW study of chiropractic was conducted with the assistance of 48 outside consultants, and every effort was made to insure that the results were "unbiased, impartial conclusions." National chiropractic organizations submitted materials and appeared before the investigating committee. On the basis of the findings, HEW concluded:

> "Chiropractic theory and practice are not based upon the body of basic knowledge related to health, disease, and health care that has been widely accepted by the scientific community. Moreover, irrespective of its theory, the scope and quality of chiropractic education do not prepare the practitioner to make an adequate diagnosis and provide appropriate treatment. Therefore, it is recommended that chiropractic services . . . not be covered in the Medicare program."[38]

Finally in 1972 Public Law 92-603 was passed to include limited services by chiropractors under Medicare beginning July 1, 1973. Section 273, "Inclusion of Chiropractors' Services Under Medicare," provides the following:

"(2) . . . a chiropractor who is licensed as such by the State (or in a State which does not license chiropractors as such, is legally authorized to perform the services of a chiropractor in the jurisdiction in which he performs such services), and who meets uniform minimum standards promulgated by the Secretary, but only for the purpose of sections 1861 (s) (1) and 1861 (s) (2) (A) and only with respect to treatment by means of manual manipulation of the spine (to correct a subluxation demonstrated by x-ray to exist) which he is legally authorized to perform by the State or jurisdiction in which such treatment is provided."

"(b) The amendments made by this section shall be effective with respect to services furnished after June 30, 1973."[39]

At the present time, therefore, Medicare covers only the chiropractor's services for manual manipulation of the spine to correct a subluxation of the spine shown in a roentgenogram. It does not pay for the roentgenogram or for any other services by the chiropractor.

Licensure

Since 1974 all of the states in the United States license chiropractors, and about 600 new licenses are issued each year. More than 20,000 chiropractors have been licensed.

An example of state law regulating chiropractors is this definition in the Texas law:

"Any person shall be regarded as practicing Chiropractic . . . who shall employ objective or subjective means without the use of drugs, surgery, X-ray therapy or radium therapy, for the purpose of ascertaining the alignment of the vertebrae of the human spine, and the practice of adjusting the vertebrae to correct any subluxation of misalignment, thereof, and charge therefore, directly or indirectly, money or other compensation."[40]

In the sections of the Texas law are such regulations as registration every year with the Texas State Board of Chiropractic Examiners; suspension of license by the State Board; one prerequisite for renewal of license—two days of "seminar, educational lectures, postgraduate course, annual convention of any State Association of Society, or regular organized Chiropractic College,"[41] violation of any part of the 1949 Chiropractic Act resulting in a misdemeanor; unprofessional conduct; and passing the basic science examination.[42] The Texas basic science examination covers "practical and theoretical chiropractic and in subjects of anatomy, physiology, symptomatology, pathology, analysis of the human spine, and hygiene and public health."[43]

Most states require four years of professional training before licensure. Thirty-four states require chiropractic students to have two years of preliminary college education beyond high school before the professional training. Some of the college courses required are biology, inorganic and organic chemistry, physiological and food chemistry, and bacteriology.

One of the aims of chiropractic education is to prepare the chiropractor to pass the basic science examination required for licensure. That examination consists of questions on anatomy, chemistry, bacteriology, diagnosis, hygiene, physiology, pathology, and public health. When these basic science examinations are given to medical students, 81.4 percent pass the examinations on the first try; when the same examinations are given to chiropractic students, 84.5 percent fail.[44]

Profile of the Chiropractor

Wrestler has indicated some characteristics of professional identification among chiropractic students:

"1. Chiropractic students perceive the chiropractor as filling a role in the healing arts which differs significantly from the medical doctor and osteopath.
"2. Chiropractic students see the role of the chiropractor, as perceived by society, as inferior to the role of the medical doctor and osteopath.
"3. Chiropractic students consider their healing art as being equivalent or superior to medicine and osteopathy and advocate a wide scope of practice and a high degree of efficacy.
"4. Chiropractic students are unclear about where to draw the boundaries of chiropractic."[45]

Evidence of this confusion about the chiropractor's role was seen in three trials by the Commonwealth of Pennsylvania. The Court barred three chiropractors from making numerous claims in advertising and told them to quit disparaging the services of medical doctors. The three chiropractors had used deceptive advertisements in newspapers. One chiropractor was told by the Court not to advertise or represent orally that his patients would "respond," that his patients could be cured by the "natural way" of chiropractic, and that medical doctors gave only temporary relief. The second chiropractor was told by the Court not to advertise or say that physical illness can be cured only by chiropractic and that pain indicated the need for a spinal analysis. The third chiropractor was told not to advertise or say that chiropractic corrected poor health, that only a chiropractor can make a person healthy, and that persons were ill because they had not visited a chiropractor.[46]

UNQUALIFIED PHYSICIANS

Specialization in medicine has reduced the number of general practitioners, concentrated physicians in large city medical centers, and produced a shortage of physicians in rural areas and in the inner city. Efforts to meet this shortage have led to the employment of medical doctors who have received their professional training in medical schools outside the United States. Many of them are well qualified, but some foreign doctors periodically take and fail the licensure examination. Masquerading under titles such as "medical technicians" or "surgical assistants," these unlicensed physicians continue to practice.

Hospitals that hire unqualified foreign physicians may include state psychiatric hospitals. Fifteen states permit employment of unlicensed physicians in state institutions. Language is sometimes a barrier between the foreign doctor and the patient, other hospital personnel, and licensed medical doctors. If unqualified physicians are practicing substandard medicine, the patient may have to pay in terms of longer hospital stays and additional medical care to correct the substandard treatment.

REFERENCES

1. Fat clinics: Ethics questioned. AMA Health Education Service, 14:1, 1974.
2. Schultz, T., and Lindeman, B.: The victimizing of desperate cancer patients. Today's Health, 51:28, 1973.
3. Masters, W. H.: Phony sex clinics—medicine's newest nightmare. Today's Health, 51:28, 1973.
4. Lindeman, B.: Cellular therapy, a shabby clinic offered rejuvenation but delivered death. Today's Health, 53:36, 1975.
5. Smith, R. L.: Strangle tales of medical imposters. Today's Health, 46:45, 1968.
6. The pain exploiters. Today's Health, 51:32, 1973.
7. Kahn, E. J.: A stamp of disapproval for these "medical" malpractitioners. Today's Health, 52:21, 1974.
8. Rice, W.: A "surgeon's" magic touch that's too good to be true. Today's Health, 52:54, 1974.
9. Rosen, S.: Beware of the "quackupuncturist" who operates for profit. Today's Health, 52:6, 1974.
10. Gwynne, P.: Acupuncture update. Today's Health, 52:16, 1974.
11. National Association of Naturopathic Physicians: Outline for Study of Services of Practitioners Performing Health Services in Independent Practice. August 1, 1968.
12. Canadian Naturopathic Association: Naturopathic Medicine in Canada. Calgary, Alberta, The Association, 1966, p. 7.
13. Ibid., p. 10.
14. Chiropractic and naturopathy. Am. J. Public Health, 60:179, 1970.
15. Smith, R. L.: Chiropractic: Science or Swindle. Today's Health, 43:56, 1965.
16. Bulletin of the Palmer College of Chiropractic, 1972-1974. Davenport, Iowa, April 1972, p. 35.
17. Independent Practitioners Under Medicare. A Report to Congress. Washington, D.C., Department of Health, Education and Welfare. December 28, 1968, p. 157.
18. HEW rejects chiropractic, op. cit.
19. Ibid.
20. Smith, R. L.: Visit to a bizarre world—chiropractic alma maters. Today's Health, 46:14, 1968.
21. Smith, R. L.: At Your Own Risk: The Case Against Chiropractic. New York, Pocket Books, Inc., 1969, pp. 101-110.
22. Smith, R. L.: Visit to a bizarre world, op. cit.
23. Smith, R. L.: At Your Own Risk, op. cit., pp. 22-23.
24. Ibid., pp. 53-68.
25. Catalog, Cleveland Chiropractic College, 1972-1974, 3700 Troost Avenue, Kansas, Missouri, 1972.
26. Catalog, Cleveland Chiropractic College, 1972-1974, 3511 W. Olympic Boulevard, Los Angeles, California, 1972.
27. Bulletin of the Palmer College of Chiropractic, 1972-1974. Davenport, Iowa, April 1972.

28. Bulletin 1971-74. Columbia Institute of Chiropractic. 261 West 71st Street, New York, New York, 1971.
29. Logan College of Chiropractic Catalog 73-74-75. 7701 Florissant Road, St. Louis, Missouri, 1973.
30. Los Angeles College of Chiropractic, Bulletin 1971-1972-1973. 920 East Broadway, Glendale, California, 1971.
31. Bulletin 71-73, National College of Chiropractic, 200 East Roosevelt Road, Lombard, Illinois, 1971-1973.
32. Northwestern College of Chiropractic. Catalog 1972-1973. 2222 Park Avenue, Minneapolis, Minnesota, 1972.
33. Texas Chiropractic College. Catalog. 1972-1974. 5912 Spencer Highway, Pasadena, Texas, 1972.
34. Western States Chiropractic College. Catalog 1973-74-75. 4525 S.E. 63rd Avenue, Portland, Oregon, 1973.
35. American Medical Association: Data Sheet on Chiropractic. Chicago, The Association's Department of Investigation, 1968, p. 1.
36. Jarvis, W. T.: Chiropractic: a challenge for health education. J. Sch. Health, 44: 210, 1974.
37. HEW rejects chiropractic. Today's Health, 47:54, 1969.
38. Chiropractic and naturopathy, op. cit.
39. Public Law 92-603, 92nd Congress, H.R. 1, Section 273, Inclusion of Chiropractor Services Under Medicare, Section 273. Washington, D.C., U.S. Government Printing Office, October 30, 1972, pp. 123-24.
40. Chiropractic Act of Texas. Rules and Regulations of the Texas Board of Chiropractic Examiners: Austin, Texas, The Board, 1949, p. 2.
41. Ibid., p. 9.
42. Sherrill, J. G. P.: Chiropractic in Texas, 1968. Unpublished Master's thesis, The University of Texas at Austin, 1970, pp. 36-45.
43. Chiropractic Act of Texas: op. cit. p. 13.
44. Smith, R. L.: Chiropractic: Science or Swindle, op. cit., p. 60.
45. Wrestler, F. A.: The Development of Professional Identification Among Chiropractic Students. Unpublished doctoral dissertation, University of Maryland, 1972. Abstract.
46. Court clamps down on 3 chiropractors' ads. Consumer Reports, 38:458, 1973.
47. Lawsuits: A growing nightmare for doctors and patients. U.S. News & World Report, 78:53, 1975.

SUPPLEMENTAL READINGS

American Chiropractic Association: Planning a Career in Chiropractic, Chiropractic's White Paper on the Health, Education, and Welfare Secretary's Report: Independent Practitioners Under Medicare. Des Moines, Iowa, The Association, 1969.

Ballantine, H. T.: Medicine and Chiropractic. Proceedings, Third National Congress on Medical Quackery. Chicago, American Medical Association, 1966.

Jelley, H. M., and Hermann, R. O.: The American Consumer: Issues and Decisions. New York, Gregg Division, McGraw-Hill Book Company, 1973.

Kahn, E. J.: Fraud. New York, Harper & Row Publishers, 1973.

McTaggart, A. C.: The Health Care Dilemma, Boston, Holbrook Press, Inc., 1971.

Margolius, S.: The Responsible Consumer. Public Affairs Pamphlet No. 453, New York, Public Affairs Committee, 1971.

Palmer, D. D.: Textbook of the Science, Art and Philosophy of Chiropractic, Founded on Tone. Portland, Oregon, Portland Printing House Company, 1910, republished 1966.

Robillard, E.: A Survey of Chiropractic. Proceedings, Third National Congress on Medical Quackery. Chicago, American Medical Association, 1966.

Sabatier, J. A.: Chiropractic—Slide Film Documentary. Proceedings, Third National Congress on Medical Quackery. Chicago, American Medical Association, 1966.

Wilson, F., and Neuhauser, D.: Health Services in the United States. Cambridge, Ballinger, 1973.

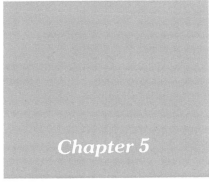

Chapter 5

HEALTH ADVERTISING—
TRUTH OR FALSEHOOD?

A N emergency respirator called "Res-Q-Aire" was seized recently by the federal Food and Drug Administration because of its danger to the user's health. The Res-Q-Aire was advertised as "easy to use, inexpensive, lightweight, medically approved." A nonprofit bio-medical engineering and testing organization released a report of a study branding Res-Q-Aire as ineffective and dangerous. More than 40,000 Res-Q-Aires have been sold. How many lives have been lost because would-be rescuers used the Res-Q-Aire on victims needing mouth-to-mouth resuscitation will never be known.[1] This example does illustrate that the consumer cannot blindly accept all of the claims made in advertisements for health products and services.

More than $17 billion are spent on advertising each year in the United States. At least 1600 advertising messages reach each American daily by such media as television, newspapers, radio, magazines, and mail. The cost of advertising headache remedies for one year may be more than $19 million (Alka-Seltzer) or more than $17 million (Bayer aspirin), excluding the cost of radio advertising.

Advertising may be defined as the printed, spoken, written, or pictured representation of a product, service, person, or organization to influence sales, get endorsements, or secure votes by an identified sponsor. The advertising industry is found not only on Madison Avenue, New York City, but also in every community where there is a newspaper, radio or television station, or an advertising agency.

DEVELOPMENT OF HEALTH ADVERTISING

Advertising of health products and services in the United States can be traced to 1708 when the first patent medicine advertisement appeared in a Boston newspaper. "Daffy's Elixir Salutis" was advertised to do wonders for its users and cost four shillings and six pence per half pint. Other packaged patent medicines shipped from England to merchants from Boston to Charleston were advertised by grocers, printers, postmasters, and apothecaries. To patent a nostrum required revealing its ingredients. American apothecaries not only imitated the imported patent medicine bottles but also marketed their own recipes of British brands. Most nostrums were unpatented and withheld their ingredients with the utmost secrecy. All brands, patented or not, were listed as "patent medicines" in advertisements.

American apothecaries built a flourishing trade in patent medicines during the American Revolution when trade was discontinued with England. After the war, American patent medicines were widespread and cheaper than their British counterparts and were sought by patriots eager to rid themselves of un-American remedies. Formulas of patent medicines, once found in British pharmocopeias, were now published for use by any American wholesale or retail druggist. The first patent medicine in the United States was patented in 1796, had an American eagle on the wrapper, and claimed to cure yellow fever, jaundice, dysentery, dropsy, and "female complaints." Later, the maker of one nostrum obtained a patent under the guise of another name but with the same ingredients as a popular nostrum already on the market.

Patent medicines thrived during the early nineteenth century because the nostrum makers advertised that their nostrums were easier means of curing ailments than the extreme bleeding and purging done by physicians. Because of the dissection of cadavers for anatomic study and the use of male physicians in obstetric cases, a steady antagonism and suspicion grew between the physician and the public.

Patent medicines, nostrums, and quacks were readily accepted by the public. Syrups and lozenges became the chief advertised nostrums when tuberculosis, typhoid, typhus, yellow fever, and cholera became prevalent from 1815 to 1835. Pills for biliousness or dyspepsia were much desired because the American diet consisted of potatoes and bread, salt-cured meats, and lard-fried foods. Fresh fruits, vegetables, and milk were lacking in urban diets.

The patent medicine merchant developed a national market, went directly to consumers, used psychologic means to entice customers, and had vivid and straightforward advertising. Newspapers were the main media of advertising the patent medicines, even in small communities with a weekly gazette. In 1858, one newspaper advertised a list of more than 500 patent medicines. Throughout the nineteenth century, advertising of patent medicines topped other advertised products. As the size and number of newspapers grew, it was not uncommon for a nostrum owner to spend a $100,000 on advertising his nostrum in one year. By the end of the nineteenth century at least a million dollars had been spent advertising Lydia E. Pinkham's Vegetable Compound.

Each owner of a nostrum had a trademark or trademarks to identify his nostrum or nostrums. These trademarks, protected by federal statute, were highly marketable commodities, even though the nostrum formula changed or the diseases for which the nostrum was advertised varied. Trademarks of patent medicines were sold and bought on the scale of mills and railroads.

Fortunes were amassed by owners of patent medicines. Many of these patent medicines were owned by major medicine manufacturers, who during the Civil War protested a federal tax on patent medicines. By 1906, the number of patent medicines numbered between 30,000 and 50,000 in the United States. The manufactured value of patent medicines was more than $75 million. Between 1902 and 1912 sales of patent medicines boomed so much that the total production of patent medicine had increased 60 percent.

Self-dosing with patent medicines grew because the disease killers of the late nineteenth century were still in evidence in 1900. The level of education among practicing physicians was low, particularly in pharmacology. Nostrum makers placed articles about the therapeutic properties of their products in medical journals and sent reprints of articles to physicians. New nostrums had scientific-sounding titles and complex formulas. The user of the patent medicine found enough information attached to the package or container for the patent medicine to discourage him from visiting a physician.

The nostrum makers exploited the advances of the physical sciences and fraudulently used biologic achievements. Following the discovery of radium by the Curies, a patent medicine, "radium impregnated," was advertised as a cure for cancer. The patent medicine was an acid solution of quinine sulfate with alcohol added. However, medical and pharmaceutical knowledge began to reach the practicing physician so that he could expose the quack.

Prevention of suffering and death was the main thrust of the early advertisements for patent medicines. From 1920, advertising aimed at the well-being and health of the customer. Advertisers tried to arouse visions of a happy American family, of superabundant leisure, of many material possessions, of romantic love, of attractiveness to the opposite sex, and of security and happiness within the home. Since health was a fundamental concern, proprietary medicines, foods, vitamins, mineral elements, soft drinks, and mouthwashes were advertised to promote good health.

The advertisements for Listerine exemplify the change in advertising. During the late nineteenth century, Listerine was marketed as a proprietary medicine as the "best antiseptic for internal and external use." In

1921, the focus of Listerine advertising was halitosis, which was advertised as a social disaster. Also, Listerine was advertised to ward off colds and sore throats, pneumonia, and other illnesses.

Other advertising for proprietary products aimed at acid indigestion, athlete's foot, body odor, dry skin, coffee nerves, sandpaper hands, dandruff, and underarm odor, to name a few. By 1934, the advertising for many products concentrated chiefly on health, happiness, and social acceptance.

Direct radio advertising by major medicine proprietors became one of the boom industries of the 1920's and 1930's. Some of the proprietary owners had their own radio stations. The quackery given in these radio broadcasts could be stopped only by the Federal Radio Commission's refusal to renew the quack's radio license.

The advent of television made it possible to combine audio and visual advertising. While listening to the hard-sell spoken word, the viewer saw headache remedies race from stomach to brain, intestines spurred into action by laxatives, and skin lotions used to create beautiful skin. "Hidden persuaders" to motivate buying were used by advertisers to sell proprietary drugs. The public, the American Medical Association, the Better Business Bureau, and members of Congress brought pressure on the Federal Trade Commission (FTC) to act firmly against proprietary advertisers. Weight-reducing and arthritis-rheumatism remedies, shampoos, antacids, and baldness cures were some of the advertised products against which the FTC campaigned.

Consumer complaints about television and radio commercials increased, particularly after the quiz show scandals in which one of the major programs had been sponsored by a proprietary manufacturer. The National Association of Broadcasters banned actors in drug commercials from wearing white coats. Also, the Association barred stations from displaying the seal of approval of its Code Board if the commercials promoted feminine hygiene products and hemorrhoid remedies.

Patent Medicines and the Rise of Consumerism

At the end of the nineteenth century newspapers and most magazines welcomed advertisements of patent medicines with no attempt to question the claims made, but the *Popular Science Monthly* and the *Ladies' Home Journal* were hostile to nostrum advertisers. Specific information concerning patent medicines and nostrums became available from investigations of the Council on Pharmacy and Chemistry of the American Medical Association, state chemists, and scientists writing in drug journals. Some newspapers revealed the hazards of patent medicines, and the *Ladies' Home Journal* broadened its attack on quackery. *Colliers* had a series written by Samuel Hopkins Adams who reserved his bitterest attack for catarrh powders containing cocaine and for soothing syrups with opium in their formulas. Adams also attacked painkillers with excessive amounts of acetanilid. For the first time, manufacturers of patent medicines were worried that federal legislation would control their nostrums. Their chief source of worry was Harvey Washington Wiley who was the scientific adviser to the Senate committee and chief drafts-man of the 1906 Pure Food and Drug Act.

One of the fervent attackers of radio advertising by quacks was *Hygeia,* the forerunner of *Today's Health,* published by the American Medical Association. Another critic was the director of the New York Tubercu-losis and Health Association, as well as periodicals such as *Nation* and *New Republic.*

Consumer's Research was organized to provide members and the public with information about the quality of products. Products were tested scientifically and described to paying members, but even more vigorous propaganda against health advertising was needed.

In 1935 the "guinea pig" muckrakers started their vigorous campaign against health advertising and worthless products. Hazards to health by many drugs, patent medicines, quack cures, and cosmetics were vividly described in such books as Kallett and Schlink's, *100,000,000 Guinea Pigs;* Phillip's, *Skin Deep: Truth About Beauty Aids—Safe and Harmful;* Schlink's, *Eat, Drink and Be Wary;* and Palmer and Greenberg's, *Facts and Frauds in Woman's Hygiene.* These muckrakers showed the Ameri-can public that any person who wanted to enter the food and drug busi-ness could experiment on the consumer and that the advertising copy-writer was not a physician. Manufacturers and advertising agencies, both large and small, were attacked. The Food and Drug Administra-tion, the Post Office Department, the American Medical Association, and the Federal Trade Commission were condemned for their pro-cedures in permitting the sale of worthless health products. The product itself, its advertising, its means of sales through the mails, and its labeling were exposed by the muckrakers.

With all the scientific discoveries to promote health, the American public, in mid-1950's, became aware that many forms of quackery still existed. Subtle in advertising, the quacks dealt with human ailments about which medical knowledge was limited and regulatory authority was untested. Medical mail frauds reached high proportions in 1957. The quacks, naturopaths, device promoters, food faddists, radicals in politics and religion, anti-fluoridationists, and the National Health Federation convinced a wide segment of the American public that physicians, phar-maceutical manufacturers, and the FDA and FTC officials were the ones endangering the health of Americans. The result was the com-bined efforts of government, medicine, and business to sound the alarm against quackery. The National Better Business Bureau issued bulle-tins on quack products such as obesity drugs, royal jelly rejuvenators, bust developers, cold remedies, arthritis gadgets, and a polio prevention scheme. The American Medical Association responded to the alarming increase in quackery by providing the public with exhibits, movies, pamphlets, and articles in *Today's Health.* Muckraking journalists, voluntary health organizations such as the American Cancer Society, and successful victories by the FDA stopped the Hoxsey cancer activities, food faddists, arthritis remedies, krebiozen, and other quacks and their products. The National Congresses on Medical Quackery (1961, 1963, and 1966) revealed how extensive was quackery in the United States.

Nostrum Makers and Government Regulation

The most powerful force against nostrums was the 1906 Pure Food and Drugs Act. Controls to be placed over patent medicines were extensively debated at a Congressional hearing. The Senate bill with stringent controls did not pass. Instead, a bill with a moderate set of nostrum controls was passed. At that time Upton Sinclair's novel, *The Jungle,* made its shocking disclosure of the meat industry and the necessity of a pure food law. This novel forced the House to bring forth a bill with more stringent controls over nostrums than the Senate bill. The House and Senate Conference reconciled their differences, and the provisions regulating nostrums emerged stronger than they had been in either bill. The result was the Pure Food and Drugs Act which required the patent medicine makers to indicate on the label the presence and amount of alcohol, chloral hydrate, the opiates, acetanilid, and other drugs in nostrums. Other ingredients did not need to be named on the label unless the maker of the patent medicine advertised other ingredients. Also, the law indicated that the label could not contain claims that were false or misleading. The Pure Food and Drugs Act of 1906 did not reduce self-medication but did try to make self-medication safer.

The narcotic content of patent medicines was at first voluntarily reduced. After the enactment of the Harrison Narcotic Act of 1914, the amount of narcotics in patent medicines was drastically eliminated. The amount of alcohol in patent medicines also was reduced because the Commissioner of Internal Revenue taxed makers of patent medicines in which alcohol was an ingredient. Patent medicines with a high alcoholic content were being purchased by those consumers with a thirst for alcohol.

To attract customers, the makers of patent medicines used "before" and "after" in their advertising. Many of the labels of patent medicines changed to such an extent that the label on the manufacturer's product not only had a new title but also had new ingredients. Critics of patent medicines showed these "before" and "after" labels to customers.

Many nostrum manufacturers continued to defy the Pure Food and Drugs Act. Often the nostrum maker would use the phrase, "Guaranteed under the Pure Food and Drugs Act," implying that the federal government endorsed the nostrum. Advertising of false claims of nostrums continued, particularly therapeutic claims. Dr. Johnson's Mild Combination Treatment for Cancer, an assortment of tablets and liquids, became the test case as to therapeutic claims. When the federal government sued the manufacturer because of the false therapeutic claims, the Supreme Court agreed with the nostrum maker's attorneys that the Pure Food and Drugs Act did not forbid false curative promises in advertising of nostrums. This decision forced Congress to pass an amendment to the Pure Food and Drugs Act declaring an article misbranded if the curative or therapeutic effect of the article or its ingredients was false and fraudulent. However, this amendment still did not deter the nostrum makers and their claims.

Journalists, physicians, scientists, and officials enforcing the Pure Food and Drugs Act tried to eliminate quackery, false claims, and patent medicines, but finally conceded that patent medicines were increasing at the rate of 200 a year. Despite legislation about labeling, many buyers of nostrums read only the advertisements in their newspapers and did not look at the labels on the containers.

From 1906 until after World War I no new federal legislation was enacted to control labeling of nostrums. The case of the federal government against the manufacturer of the nostrum, Microbe Killer, showed that fraud could be deduced from a nostrum's label. The label indicated that this product could cure measles, malaria, worms, consumption, yellow fever, small pox, leprosy, and headache. Federal authorities seized 539 wooden boxes and 322 pasteboard cartons of Microbe Killer which was to sell for $5166 but could be made at a cost of $25.82. The mixture was 99 percent tap water and 1.0 percent sulfuric acid. The jury condemned the nostrum's labels as fraudulent. From that time on, a steady campaign was waged against patent medicines, their labels, and claims for curing various diseases. Campaigns were launched against throat and lung patent medicines, kidney and liver remedies, mineral waters having "cure-all" claims, male rejuvenators, and other viscious nostrums. Concoctions to cure venereal diseases were supposedly driven off the market. Many patent medicines had to modify their labeling

Since mechanical devices were not drugs, these devices could claim cures for dread diseases. Also, quack concoctions for weight reduction were not included in the law. As long as the nostrum makers did not place therapeutic claims on the labels of cosmetic preparations, these preparations were not in conflict with the law. Many powerful poisons that were not included in the Pure Food and Drugs Act were placed in these cosmetic preparations.

During the Franklin Delano Roosevelt administration, further attempts were made to regulate quack products, patent medicines, cosmetics, and dangerous drugs. In the years following the passage of the

Pure Food and Drugs Act, officials of the FDA became aware of the many loopholes in the law. The first proposed legislation was the Tugwell bill. Regulations about labeling on drugs, medicinal ingredients in proprietary medicines, medicines containing narcotics, dangerous drugs, quack products and remedies, false advertising, and self-dosing included in advertising and on labels were some features of the Tugwell bill. Also, the FDA could inspect factories where proprietary drugs were manufactured. Opposition was tremendous, but the FDA continued its fight for the Tugwell bill. One means was its Chamber of Horrors—an exhibit of labels, advertisements, posters, and bottles of quack products and death certificates of persons using the quack products. The Tugwell bill was defeated.

Revisions of the Tugwell bill followed and were defeated. Often groups interested in consumer protection joined with medicine makers because of the wording of the revisions. One of the issues in these revised bills was the substitution of the Federal Trade Commission for the Food and Drug Administration as the agency to supervise food, drug, and cosmetic advertising. Another issue was to weaken the FDA's multiple seizure authority. Finally, a much-patched pure food and drug bill was passed by the Senate. When the bill came before the House subcommittee, events took a turn for the better. When the substitute food and drug bill was brought into the House, it gave sole control of food, drug, and cosmetic advertising to the Federal Trade Commission. This substitute food and drug bill passed and spurred state legislatures to pass more vigorous food and drug acts.

In 1938, a more comprehensive food and drug bill appeared before the House of Representatives. The result was the Wheeler-Lea Act which gave the FTC control over advertising. Also, advertisers who could be proved guilty of fraud or who advertised dangerous products could be told to cease and desist their false advertising. Fines for guilty advertisers were removed from the Act. With the advertising issue of the food and drug bill settled, the comprehensive food and drug bill had a chance to survive.

As the new food and drug bill came to the attention of Congress, deaths from Elixir Sulfanilamide were being reported. In the preparation of this medicine, the chemist testing the concoction had failed to prove the safety of the medicine. Also, this Elixir did not contain alcohol and was misbranded. The FDA tracked down 99.2 percent of all Elixir Sulfanilamide and reported the deaths of 107 persons. The public urged Congress to plug loopholes in the food and drug law.

In 1938, Congress passed the Food, Drug, and Cosmetic Act. The definition of misbranding of proprietary medicines was stronger than in the 1906 Act. False and misleading labeling was banned. False labeling included omission of warnings in circumstances where medication might be hazardous. Dangerous drugs were outlawed, and the formulas for nonofficial drugs were to be disclosed. All active ingredients in medications had to be placed upon the label. The quantity and dosage of narcotics and hypnotic drugs had to be stated. Antiseptics had to be germicidal. New drugs could not be marketed until they were proven safe. Quack products and medicines shipped by mail by "doctors" were included in the law, and the FDA's seizures and procedures against quacks were strengthened because the agency was now authorized to seek injunctions against them.

When the Food, Drug, and Cosmetic Act became effective, World War II forced the FDA into national emergency responsibilities and provided quacks with new opportunities. They turned to promotion of mechanical devices, obesity products, pain-killers, abortifacient pastes, laxatives, and cures for alcoholism. Hazardous devices such as breast pumps, nipple shields, electric insoles, respirators, trusses, catheters, ear droppers, and massagers were taken off the market by the FDA. Nostrum makers disguised their nostrums as prescription items, since this loophole existed in the Food, Drug, and Cosmetic Law.

After World War II, prescription drugs dominated in sales due to manufacture of penicillin, other antibiotics, synthetic vitamins, new vaccines, antihistamines, hormone-like compounds, tranquilizers, and other therapeutic agents. Pharmaceutical manufacturers entered the self-medication field, advertising over-the-counter drugs through radio, television, magazines, and the press. The leaders in sales were analgesics, mainly aspirin and compounds containing aspirin, laxatives, vitamins, cold and cough preparations, antacids and stomach sweeteners, antiseptics, and liniments. The FDA insisted that possible hazards of the commonest remedy must be listed on the label. Some of these cautions were (1) to seek medical care if pain persists, (2) not to take a laxative when the customer has an abdominal pain, (3) to avoid driving a car when taking antihistamines because they may cause drowsiness, and (4) to keep aspirin out of the reach of children.

The problem of controlling the sale of hazardous drugs, including barbiturates resulted in the passage of the Durham-Humphrey Amendment in 1951. In the original draft, three categories of prescription drugs could not be refilled without specific authorization of the physician: habit-forming drugs, new drugs released for marketing by the FDA but limited to prescription sale, and drugs to be used only under supervision of a physician and so designated by the FDA. The third category of drugs would draw a sharp line between prescription and self-medication drugs. Congress removed from the FDA the authority to determine prescription and nonprescription drugs, but the FDA continued to fight to make self-medication efficacious as well as safe.

The Durham-Humphrey Act proved to be difficult to enforce because some pharmaceutical manufacturers and pharmacists wanted to move many prescription drugs to over-the-counter drugs. The majority of pharmacists wanted prescription drugs released slowly as over-the-counter drugs. In this way, the pharmacist could tell his customers about warnings on labels, caution his customers against excessive purchases, and supervise self-medication. However, the Proprietary Medicine Manufacturers and Dealers Association, drug wholesalers, some pharmaceutical manufacturers, and grocery associations tried to defeat state laws growing out of the Durham-Humphrey Act. Unfortunately, this Act did not completely stop the illegal possession of barbiturates, amphetamines, and other powerful hypnotic drugs.

A near-disaster from thalidomide led to the passage of the Kefauver-Harris Drug Amendments to the Food, Drug, and Cosmetic Act of 1938 by both Houses of Congress in 1962. These amendments improved the FDA's control over the marketing and promotion of prescription drugs. Although these amendments attempted to require the same inspection of plants of manufacturers of proprietary products as of those for prescription drugs, this effort failed. Control of advertising for prescription drugs was placed under the jurisdiction of the FDA. Each advertisement had to present truthfully each drug's effectiveness, side effects, and contraindications. The new proof-of-efficacy premarketing standard applied to both over-the-counter and prescription drugs. However, as revealed in Chapters 1 and 2, quacks and food faddists continued to sell over-the-counter drugs and promote them by all types of advertising.

Proprietary Medicine Manufacturers and Dealers Association

In 1881, the Proprietary Medicine Manufacturers and Dealers Association was formed. This group represented the owners of nostrums and protested the printing of formulas of nostrums by persons or groups other than Association members. The Association sought to control the use of trademarks and to prohibit counterfeiting of labels. It took quick action when Congress or state legislatures proposed any measure restricting patent medicines or controlling advertising of them. By 1915 members of the Proprietary Association were producing 80 percent of the patent medicines.

The American Pharmaceutical Association established a special commission on proprietary medicines which consented to meet with a committee of the Proprietary Association. This commission had devised "Minimum Requirements with Which Proprietary Remedies Should Comply in Order to Render Them Safe for Direct Sales to the General Public." Narcotics were not to be given to children and were not to exceed the Harrison Law requirements if the proprietary medicines were for adults. Alcohol was to be kept to the minimum needed to keep the active ingredients in solution from freezing. No false statements concerning therapeutic effects were to be found on the package. However, the Proprietary Association was less stringent than the American Pharmaceutical Association as to advertising and labeling. The Proprietary Association agreed that no patent medicine could be advertised as a cure for a disease or condition generally recognized as incurable.

From the time the Pure Food and Drugs Act became effective, the Proprietary Association had to urge its members to improve the standards. The Association and its patent medicine makers were being criticized by magazines like *Collier's* and by a strongly developing retail trade. Legislation restricting the patent medicine makers and removing secrecy were being enacted. The influence of the Association had waned.

Nostrums Sold by Mail and the Post Office

From the beginning of the twentieth century, the Post Office Department has attacked advertising of nostrums. A test letter would be sent to the nostrum maker by postal inspectors who would request information about the maker's cures for epilepsy, cancer, deafness, blindness, the drug habit, lost manhood, failing womanhood, and the tobacco habit. In 1904, the Postmaster General issued two fraud orders to two companies which had sent pamphlets advertising cures for lost manhood, urinary trouble, and kidney disorders through the mail. Nostrums were mailed to a customer upon receipt of the purchaser's money order. Even though the nostrum makers abandoned their businesses, they were shortly back in business wiser in ways to avoid any fraud orders of the Postmaster General. Again, advertisements of nostrums to cure lost manhood and weak kidneys were placed in newspapers and magazines. The customer answering the advertisement was urged to buy the Man Medicine from the nostrum maker so that his sexual strength would improve. Since most men did not want their ailments known by friends and families, they indicated to the nostrum maker that the Man Medicine would be paid in cash on delivery. The Man Medicine would be a formula that any druggist could fill. Often Man Medicine was sent to men whose names were on a "sucker list," even though the recipients had placed no orders for the cure. A fraud order was issued by the Postmaster General. The nostrum maker was fined $5,000. A list of a half million men who had received advertised nostrums through the mail was turned over to the government. This case revealed that many nostrum owners bought their wares from ethical drug producers, whose names never appeared on the nostrums. These manufacturers supplied the advertising literature used by the nostrum distributor and aided him to stay in business.

With the increasing availability of over-the-counter drugs, the quack could use these drugs and his cures for worthless therapeutic claims advertised by mail direct to the customer. The quacks had cures for cancer, diabetes, and rheumatism; nostrums to develop the female breasts and improve male virility; and remedies for all types of illness. As in the Man Medicine case, the Post Office Department continued to issue fraud orders to any quack who did not abandon his mail-order sales and advertising until the Supreme Court ruled that the Post Office Department had to bring quacks and their products before impartial judges selected by the Civil Service Commission. These judges based their decision upon the testimony of witnesses for the Post Office Department and the quacks. During the hearing clever quacks would employ attorneys who could use stalling tactics that would permit the quack to continue to advertise and sell his product through the mail. Later, the Post Office Department was forced to prove that the quack had deliberately intended to promote a fraudulent product. Thus, the quack could seek counsel from doctors of questionable reputation and be assured his miraculous cure had therapeutic value. When testifying at the Post Office Department's hearing, the quack could rely on his experts and claim innocence, since the Post Office Department had to prove that the defendant had knowingly and intentionally sold a fraudulent product. The quack promoting arthritis remedies, vitamins and other nutritional schemes, and drugs and devices for weight reduction soon learned how to avoid a fraud case.

The test case was Kelpidine case. Kelpidine was dried seaweed, extensively advertised by its promoter, Joseph Pinkus, as a weight reducer. Nothing in the labeling referred to Kelpidine as a reducing agent, regardless of what the advertising promised. None of the advertising conveyed to the customer that he would reduce his food intake by using Kelpidine. Rather, the advertising promised that the customer could eat as he usually did. A fraud order against Pinkus was ordered by the Post Office Department.

Other mail-order promoters had frequent contacts with Post Office Department attorneys. In 1915 the Department won a criminal case against the maker of a quack mechanical device promoted and sold by mail. When postal inspectors have won their cases, the quacks have turned from one cure to another, knowing that medical care for conditions such as cancer, obesity, and rheumatism is not fully understood by the public. Even though scientific evidence has been reaching the courts, the Post Office Department and Postal Service has had to wage a steady battle with quacks advertising nostrums through the mail. As long as American consumers know little about mail-order quacks and continue buying their products and services, mail-order quackery will be a thriving business.

Labeling of Nostrums and the Food and Drug Administration

To ban testimonials in advertising, the Food and Drug Administration spent more than $75,000 in ten years of hard work on the B&M case. B&M, a mixture of turpentine and ammonia, was originally a horse liniment. The B&M labeling, however, claimed it could cure pneumonia, bronchitis, hay fever, rheumatism, peritonitis, neuritis, varicose veins, sprains, cancer, blood poisoning, asthma, tuberculosis, and other diseases and ailments. At a time when tuberculosis was prevalent, B&M was advertised as an external remedy to be rubbed on the chest to rid the lungs of tuberculosis. Testimonials from users of B&M were gathered by the nostrum owner and published in pamphlets and newspapers. The Boston health commissioner asserted that B&M's owner violated state law by "false and misleading" advertising. Although the government called reputable physicians as expert witnesses to show that rubbing B&M on the chest did not reach tuberculosis in the lungs and showed that B&M's owner had no preparation to practice medicine when prescribing a cure for tuberculosis, the maker of B&M produced the testimonials from users and was able to convince the jury that he believed B&M had the power to produce the intended effect of curing tuberculosis. The government lost the case.

Several years later, the FDA seized shipments of B&M and charged adulteration and misbranding. In the second court case of B&M, the nostrum owner compiled new testimonials, secured services of a minister-physician and pharmacist, and used the owner of a private research center to validate the effectiveness of B&M as a cure for tuberculosis. At that time, the FDA's use of multiple seizures to suppress nostrums had been an indispensable legal weapon. The B&M attorney was able to stop seizures of B&M by the FDA until a test case could be tried. When the B&M case came to trial, the B&M attorney attempted to persuade the jury that no one had been guilty of fraud. Testimonials were given that B&M could cure tuberculosis. However, the government had results of clinical trials using B&M on tuberculosis patients, testimony from medical specialists, and laboratory evidence from noted pharmacologists; introduced evidence from physicians treating men and women who gave testimonials; and presented death certificates and hospital records of persons who gave testimonials but did not have tuberculosis—all showing the worthlessness of B&M. The jury found that the maker of B&M had violated an amendment to the Pure Food and Drugs Act in claiming a cure by a fraudulent product.

Test court cases included Colusa Natural Oil, a nostrum sold to treat psoriasis, eczema, leg ulcers, and athlete's foot. The owner of this nostrum was one of many antagonists who tried to test the legality of the Food, Drug, and Cosmetic Act of 1938. Others tried to circumvent the law pertaining to labeling, promotional literature, or ingredients. The FDA attacked misleading labeling by pseudomedical promoters and the addition of worthless ingredients to proprietary medicines by quacks who claimed them to be therapeutic.

The quack adopted new approaches to reach the public after he was forced to eliminate false claims from labels. The quacks became salesmen, talking to informal groups, booming their sales pitch over public address systems, providing free lectures, or going from door to door. The FDA inspectors used tape recorders to collect evidence in their attempts to reduce the false claims of food faddists, health lecturers, and "specialists" with cures. The quack selling drugs and devices for self-treatment moved into chronic health conditions such as arthritis. However, the field of quackery which gained the most financial reward for the quack was food faddism (Chapter 2).

As the FDA moved to curtail the activities of quacks, clinics appeared as treatment centers that appealed to the sick and frightened. Chiropractors, naturopaths, and unscrupulous physicians and osteopaths ran the clinics or hired operators to diagnose and treat customers. Mechanical devices (Chapter 1) and pseudodrug products such as dried vegetables and glandular extracts were means of attracting customers. When the FDA won cases in the courts, the quacks were given short prison sentences and small fines, despite the FDA's careful preparation of its cases. Also, the FDA was handicapped by lack of funds and inspectors.

In 1948, the Food and Drug Administration won its case against the Kaadt brothers after a long investigation. These two physicians knew not only that there was no cure for diabetes, but that insulin and a restricted diet free of sugar were necessary in the control of diabetes. The Kaadt brothers, Charles and Peter, founded the Kaadt Diabetic Institute where they discredited the accepted medical care of a diabetic and promoted their miraculous medicine as a substitute for insulin, diet, and medical care. The medicine was sold by mail and without any examination of the patient. When the medicine was chemically analyzed, it contained saltpeter dissolved in vinegar. When the younger brother, Peter Kaadt, took over the business, he closed the Institute, stopped prescribing by mail, did not treat children, and destroyed pamphlets advertising the miraculous medicine, but continued to dispense medicine by individual prescription. He advocated that diabetes was a disease of the sympathetic nervous system, that vinegar and saltpeter stimulated the digestive system, and that insulin, diet, and exercise were wrong in the care of the diabetic. Charles and Peter Kaadt were each fined $7000 and sent to prison for four years.

Mechanical quackery boomed when the FDA halted other forms of quackery. Often the mechanical devices were being used by chiropractors, osteopaths, and licensed physicians. The mechanical device might be used by the quack in a clinic or laboratory and sold to the customer for home use (Chapter 1). Two significant antiquackery cases won by the FDA were the Drown case and the Micro-Dynameter. The Drown case not only made the public more aware of mechanical quackery but also prohibited mechanical devices from distribution in interstate commerce. The Micro-Dynameter was proved dangerous because of its promoter's claims that the device could diagnose numerous diseases which it did not diagnose.

Advertising of Nostrums and the Federal Trade Commission

While the FDA was waging its battle against B&M, the FTC was fighting the Raladam Company for its false advertising. In 1914 the FTC was established to "investigate, publicize, and prohibit all unfair methods of competition." A year later, a delegation from the Associated Advertising Clubs of the World urged the Commission to control false and fraudulent advertising. Previously, *Printers Ink*—a spokesman for decent advertising—had proposed a Model Statute for advertising which was enacted by many states but seldom enforced. Before 1918 the Commission had issued 2000 of the first 3000 cease and desist orders to restrain false advertising. Fake advertisements for anti-fat remedies, medicines for incurable diseases, soaps, and fraudulent therapeutic devices were common.

The FTC decided to take joint action against the advertiser and the publisher of the advertisement for an obesity cream, Reducine. The advertisements appeared in *True Romances*. The advertisements of Reducine stressed that excess fat was dissolved away by application of the obesity cream. The FTC issued to the Reducine maker and the publisher of *True Romances* cease and desist orders but delayed its action so that agencies of self-regulation might promote "truth in advertising."

Self-regulation involved the National Better Business Bureau (NBBB), which had assumed leadership to develop codes regulating advertising behavior. Among the codes was the agreement that the FTC would not act against a publisher until self-regulation had had its chance. The NBBB issued a series of bulletins critical of the advertising for obesity cures, health foods, nostrums for goiter and female weakness, external health and beauty appliances, bust developers, baldness, rupture, deafness, piles, rheumatism, optical remedies, and tobacco cures, among others. At the top of the list of the bulletins from the NBBB was the fat-reducer, Reducine. When advertisers erred, the FTC issued cease and desist orders.

The critical court decision concerned the advertising of a weight-reducing remedy, Marmola. Marmola contained dried thyroid glands of various animals and did cause obese people to lose weight. Some pharmaceutical companies were glad to sell desiccated thyroid medication and to give scientific advice to the nostrum maker as to dosage. Also, obesity was not a disease, so cures for obesity were not considered for investigation by the FDA. The formula for Marmola changed from year to year but did contain laxatives. Advertisements urged men and women to use Marmola since the popular fad was to appear lithe, slim, slender, and beautiful.

In 1928 the FTC challenged Marmola's advertising such as, fat people suffer from underactive thyroid. The FTC had testimony from officials of the FDA, medical professors, and the head of the Bureau of Investigation, American Medical Association as to the dangerous effects of Marmola. In 1929 the FTC issued an order for the Marmola owner to stop advertising Marmola as a harmless cure for obesity. The owner petitioned a circuit court to remove the order. The FTC fought the petition and sought an injunction to forbid the Marmola owner to continue the false advertising. The court gave its judgment to Marmola and canceled the FTC's order. The FTC appealed the decision to the Supreme Court. The Court rigidly interpreted the law as to the FTC's "sphere of usefulness" in controlling abuses in advertising, thus giving the FTC less power. Advertising became ruthless, and a period of muckraking swept over respectable manufactures of proprietary medicines.

After the Wheeler-Lea Act was enacted, the FTC slowly used its cease and desist orders with little effect in controlling the advertising of nostrums. In 1947 the FTC permitted the removal of possible hazards from advertising for certain laxatives, headache remedies, and other self-medication drugs. Due to this action, cases were lost by the FTC. Advertisers of proprietary drugs and quack products found there were many ways to bypass the FTC.

By 1960, neither self-regulation by the proprietary advertisers or renewed efforts of the FTC had brought about "truth" in proprietary advertising. Deodorant commercials, as well as advertisements for headache remedies, stomach sweeteners, dentifrices, dyspepsia remedies, laxatives, and cold and sinus inhalants, struck television viewers as obnoxious. A year later the FTC still had not found a way to stop false advertising of proprietary products.

Possibly the largest sum spent for advertising a proprietary product was for Hadacol, which had sales of $20 million within 22 states in one year. Advertising cost a million dollars a month and was placed in 700 daily, 4700 weekly newspapers and on 528 radio stations. As sales boomed, the advertising which had featured testimonials claiming cures for anemia, asthma, arthritis, cancer, diabetes, epilepsy, gallstones, heart trouble, tuberculosis, ulcers, and other illnesses changed to statements of "good health" and added a money-back guarantee. Testimonials came from ordinary persons like the customer and his neighbors. The advertising took on the aura of the old-time medicine show built on circus-like proportions. In addition to jokes related to sexual prowess, the promoter of Hadacol sought the sanction of orthodox medicine for his product, used all types of advertising tricks, became involved in state politics, and tried to get Hadacol classified as an "ethical proprietary."[2]

The Federal Trade Commission is authorized:

"To safeguard the consuming public by preventing the dissemination of false or deceptive advertisements of food, drugs, cosmetic and therapeutic devices, and other unfair or deceptive practices."

"To regulate packaging and labeling of certain consumer commodities so as to prevent consumer deception and facilitate value comparisons."

Complaint may be made by a consumer; a competitor; Federal, state, or municipal agencies; or the Commission itself. A letter giving facts and accompanied by evidence in possession of the complaining party is sent to the Commission. Upon receipt of an application for complaint, the Commission decides whether the complaint shall be docketed for investigation. On completion of the investigation, there may be (1) "informal settlement of the case on the respondent's assurance of discontinuance of the illegal practice; (2) issuance of a formal complaint; or (3) closing the case." If a complaint is issued by the Commission, the party so concerned is given a copy of the complaint and order. The respondent can consent to the cease and desist order without admitting violation of law. If an agreement containing a consent order is not reached, the Commission may issue its complaint. The case is heard by an administrative law judge, after testimony has been taken at public hearings. The judge issues the initial decision, which becomes the decision of the Commission at the end of 30 days unless the respondent appeals to the Commission. Violation of an order to cease and desist after it becomes final brings the offender to trial by the Government in a United States district court and a fine of $5000 for each violation. When the violation continues, each day of its continuance is a separate offense.

Dissemination of a false advertisement of a food, drug, device, or cosmetic that may be injurious to the user's health or where there is intent to defraud constitutes a misdemeanor. The convicted offender pays a fine of not more than $5000 or imprisonment of not more than six months, or both. Succeeding convictions may result in a fine of not more than $10,000 or imprisonment of not more than one year, or both.[3]

TYPES OF ADVERTISING BY QUACKS

Quacks selling health products practice deception in their advertising. In addition to using half-truths, exaggerated promises, and false claims they search for ways to outwit the law.

Photographs of clinics outfitted with all types of scientific-sounding gadgetry may be used in advertisements of mechanical quacks. Words, like "magnetism, vibrations, ionic effects, cosmic radiation, trace minerals, and organic foods" are some of the terms used in advertising. Some quacks have advertised that they are supported by research grants.

Testimonials are used in advertising today as in the past. "Regimen— the wonder drug to lose weight" was advertised by national television advertising. Regimen consisted of ammonium chloride, a diuretic, and phenylpropanolamine, an appetite depressant. The advertisement showed overweight housewives supposedly eating the foods they wanted to eat and taking Regimen. These living proofs of weight loss through

Regimen were professional actresses on near starvation diets of 500 calories daily.

A quack product may advertise in a local newspaper. "Doorbell doctors" then work neighborhoods in teams of two. One works under the guise of conducting a "health survey" and discovers the ailments of the people in a neighborhood. A week or two later, the other salesman offers a quack product to cure the surveyed people with ailments. The second salesman may reappear with other quack remedies to cure the ailments faster.

Small-time quacks may peddle door to door or send by mail dangerous drugs for cures of chronic health conditions such as epilepsy. The drug may be phenobarbital advertised as a homemade remedy.

Gadgets like the "radionic machine" are advertised to cure diseases. In the hands of a quack, certain medical equipment, such as an X-ray machine, could be especially dangerous to a patient if the X-ray machine is poorly made and operated. The naturopath, sanipractor, scientologist, and electrotherapist usually have no way of testing medical equipment they purchase and use on their victims.

The physician or hospital administrator may purchase faulty equipment because of the false claims, half-truths, or exaggerated promises of the manufacturer's advertising or his salesmen. An advertising agency may promote poorly designed and manufactured surgical and hospital equipment, not knowing that the manufacturer has not tested it adequately or has no rigid quality controls. Certain companies do extensive testing of their medical products and stress rigid quality controls in their manufacture. In other companies standards for the designing and manufacturing of medical products are inadequate or nonexistent. These products include heart pacemakers, hip pins, synthetic arteries, cobalt radiation machines, and patient monitoring systems. Surgical implants may be made from ordinary commercial grade steel causing toxic reactions within the body. Metal implants not subjected to proper tests for stress may snap inside a leg or arm and cause an electrolytic reaction. Synthetic blood vessels may break down when grafted into the human body. Artificial heart valves may cause fatal blood clots because of poor design or improper manufacture. In one study, faulty electrical equipment in hospital operating rooms caused 1200 patients to be electrocuted during 1964 and 1965.[4]

Four current types of advertising used to fleece the consumer are (1) bait and switch, (2) chain referral, (3) free gimmick, and (4) fear sell.

Bait and Switch

In bait-and-switch advertising the quack or salesman selling the quack product advertises a product which he has no intention of selling so that the customer can be switched to another product. Bait-and-switch advertising is legal in many states and is so subtle that most customers are not aware that they have been deceived. An advertisement placed in a local newspaper urges the reader to buy a food supplement sold by door-to-door salesmen and produced by a nationally known pharmaceutical company. Any of the myths promoted by food faddists may be used in the advertisement (Chapter 2). When the door-to-door salesman reaches the customer, the customer finds the food supplement offered is an off-brand product. If the customer protests, the salesman rushes to his car for another off-brand and more expensive food supplement. A discount is offered because it is the salesman's first day on the job. The salesman's volume of sales and profit are in the lesser known brand. The food supplement produced by a nationally known pharmaceutical company is never intended to be sold by the salesman, but occasionally may be sold, if the customer insists.

Phony hearing aids are sold to many elderly persons by high-pressure salesmen. A well-known reputable hearing aid will be advertised and then the salesman will substitute a shabby aid that can be made for less than one dollar. Some advertisements indicate that the hearing aid can be worn invisibly to cure any hearing problem. Sometimes a salesman of hearing aids may test the hearing of the customer in the buyer's home or pressure the customer to buy a hearing aid when the customer is totally deaf. At least 70 percent of the 500,000 persons who buy hearing aids in one year go directly to a dealer rather than to a physician.

Chain Referral

Chain-referral advertising has become such a major problem that the Postal Service has a special investigative project to handle these swindles. The customer is led to believe that he will make money by referring names of friends and relatives, as prospective customers, to the promoter of the quack product. For each acquaintance who is sold, the customer is promised a commission. The customer who agrees to participate in an advertising campaign is promised a commission. Door-to-door salesmen of products promoted by food faddists will tell prospective customers that a large percentage of the referred persons will buy the product. They have charts showing that within a few months the prospective customer can make a thousand dollars. To gain this commission, the prospective customer must sign advertising notices of the faddist's product, which the faddist will mail to persons whose names the customer sends to the faddist's headquarters. If the prospective customer indicates that he cannot afford the expensive product, the salesman convinces the customer to buy a "discounted" product to enter the advertising campaign. Seldom does the customer receive a commission for the names of acquaintances or for their purchases of the faddist's product. The salesman has the money the customer paid for the discounted product.

Free Gimmick

The free-gimmick advertising is accompanied by numerous misrepresentations and half-truths. The advertising indicates that the customer gets a food supplement worth $25 without cost if the customer subscribes to a monthly food-supplement plan. The food supplement given without cost may be worth a few dollars and may be an off-brand product. The monthly plan may be ten times more expensive than the housewife's food bill. A variation is a telephone call informing the customer that he has received a first prize in a contest which provides $100 off the purchase price of a six-month supply of food supplements. The phony $200 "regular" purchase price is $150 more than the original price. Thus, the salesman profits $50. Variations of the free-gimmick advertising are numerous: "If you can answer this question, you can have $5 worth of food supplements absolutely free" or "You can have $5 worth of free food supplements since your name has been chosen from a list of outstanding community citizens."

"Free medical examination at our clinic" is another advertising gimmick used by unscrupulous quacks. A telephone call is placed to a person in an area of a large city where there are many ill and poor. Believing the clinic to be government-operated, the person will go to the clinic. There he is told he must have an X-ray and be placed on a multiple treatment plan. The victim signs an installment contract to cover the treatments. That contract may cost $300 and is collected by having the employer deduct a sum from the person's weekly wages. If the victim does not pay, he may receive an intimidating letter on a letterhead bearing the name of some fictitious government agency.

Fear Sell

Fear-sell advertising has been promoted for centuries. Amulets were advertised to protect the wearer from diseases or accidents and were sold to rich and poor alike. The food faddist may promote a product to prevent certain illnesses, e.g., arthritis. The salesmen solicit sales by door-to-door contacts and show pictures of persons ill with arthritis. The prospective customer is led to believe he can avoid the crippling effects of arthritis by subscribing to a food-supplement plan or by buying the neatly wrapped food supplement. Usually a discount is offered for a cash sale.[5]

REFERENCES

1. Medical devices: an unhealthy situation. Consumer Reports, 35:256, 1970.
2. Young, J. H.: The Medical Messiahs. Princeton, New Jersey, Princeton University Press, 1967, pp. 13-423.
3. Office of the Federal Register. National Archives and Records Service. General Services Administration: United States Government Organization Manual, 1973-1974. Washington, D.C., U.S. Government Printing Office, 1973, pp. 469-474.
4. Medical devices: an unhealthy situation, op. cit., p. 258.

5. Magnuson, W. G.: The Dark Side of the Marketplace: the Plight of the American Consumer. Englewood Cliffs, New Jersey, Prentice-Hall, Inc., 1968, pp. 3-31.

SUPPLEMENTAL READINGS

Amstell, I. J.: What You Should Know About Advertising. Dobbs Ferry, New York, Oceana Publications, Inc., 1969.
Howard, J. A., and Sheth, J. N.: The Theory of Buyer Behavior. New York, John Wiley & Sons, Inc., 1969.
Margolius, S.: Buyer Be Wary! #382. New York, Public Affairs Committee, 1968.
Margolius, S.: The Innocent Consumer vs. the Exploiters. New York, Trident Press, 1968.
Markin, R. J.: The Psychology of Consumer Behavior. Englewood Cliffs, New Jersey, Prentice-Hall, Inc., 1969.
Masters, D.: The Intelligent Buyer and Telltale Seller. New York, Afred A. Knopf, Inc., 1966.
Sandage, C. H.: The Promise of Advertising. Homewood, Illinois, Richard D. Irwin, Inc., 1968.
Zacher, R. V.: Advertising Techniques and Management, Revised Edition. Homewood, Illinois, Richard D. Irwin, Inc., 1967.

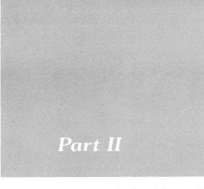

Part II

WISE CONSUMER

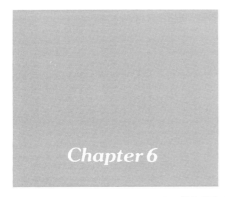

Chapter 6

HEALTH INSURANCE

THE National Health Survey revealed that American wage earners lose at least 294 million work days in a year due to illness or injury. For each worker, an average of 3.8 to 4 days have been lost each year, with the average male employee being absent fewer work days than the average employed female. Respiratory illnesses and accidents were the two leading causes of lost work days. Workers with family annual incomes of less than $3000 had more than twice the number of days of restricted activity because of illness or injury than workers with family annual incomes of more than $3000. The average American in the survey had more than twice the number of days of restricted activity compared to days of bed disability because of illness or injury. The number of bed-disability days for persons whose family incomes were less than $3000 was more than twice the average.

Physician visits were reported by the National Health Survey. Visits included consultation with a physician, either in person or by telephone, but did not include the physician's visits to his patient in a hospital. In a year, Americans have had 927 million physician visits, for an average of 4.6 visits per person. Women had more physician visits than men. Fifty percent of surveyed children and youth had at least one physician visit per year. Fourteen percent of the persons surveyed had not visited a physician in two or more years.

It has been estimated that there is an immediate need for more than 150,000 active registered nurses, 90,000 licensed practical nurses, and 70,000 medical doctors. Also, more than 250,000 hospital beds are needed, and facilities housing another 250,000 require urgent modernization. Ten percent of the medical schools may be facing imminent closing for lack of funds. At least 280,000 other health specialists and 20,000 dentists are needed.

TABLE 6-1
PERSONAL CONSUMPTION EXPENDITURES
BY TYPE OF PRODUCT
In the United States, 1971

Type of Product	Personal consumption expenditures (billions of dollars)	Percent of total
Food (including alcohol)	$136.4	20.5%
Housing	99.2	14.9
Household operation	93.6	14.1
Transportation	90.1	13.5
Clothing, accessories, and jewelry	66.9	10.1
Medical care*	50.1	7.5
Recreation	42.5	6.4
Personal business	36.1	5.4
Tobacco	11.7	1.8
Private education and research	11.1	1.7
Personal care	10.6	1.6
Religious and welfare activities	9.1	1.4
Foreign travel and remittances—net	5.2	0.8
Death expenses	2.3	0.3
Total	$664.9	100.0%

*Includes all expenses for health insurance.
Sources: United States Department of Commerce and Department of Health, Education, and Welfare.
By permission of the Health Insurance Institute, 277 Park Avenue, New York, N. Y. 10017.

In 1971, the American public spent more than $50 billion on health care. Of all personal consumption expenditures, medical care cost 7.5 percent (Table 6-1). The amount in 1971 was 155 percent more than that spent in 1961. Per capita expenditures for personal health care more than doubled when those expenditures in 1971 are compared to those in 1960 (Table 6-2). Costs of privately controlled hospital care were 246 percent more in 1971 than in 1961. In 1971, $13 billion were spent for payments of physician's services and $9 billion for medicines and appliances. Other types of medical care, excluding dental fees and net cost of health insurance, increased 105 percent between 1961 and 1971 (Table 6-3). Medical costs increased faster than any other major category of personal expense from 1967 to 1971. Hospital rates increased 61 percent, physicians' fees 30 percent, dentists' fees 27 percent, and optometric examinations and costs of eyeglasses 20 percent (Table 6-4).

The American Hospital Association reported that the cost of treating a patient in community hospitals increased 92 percent between

TABLE 6-2
RATIO OF PERSONAL CONSUMPTION EXPENDITURES FOR MEDICAL CARE TO DISPOSABLE PERSONAL INCOME AND TO TOTAL PERSONAL CONSUMPTION EXPENDITURES
In the United States
(billions of dollars)

Year	Personal consumption expenditures for medical care*	Disposable personal income	Total personal consumption expenditures	Ratio of Col. (1) of Col. (2)	Ratio of Col. (1) to Col. (3)
	(1)	(2)	(3)	(4)	(5)
1948	$ 7.5	$189.1	$173.6	4.0%	4.3%
1950	8.5	206.9	191.0	4.1	4.5
1955	12.3	275.3	254.4	4.5	4.8
1960	18.6	350.0	325.2	5.3	5.7
1961	19.7	364.4	335.2	5.4	5.9
1962	21.4	385.3	355.1	5.6	6.0
1963	22.8	404.6	375.0	5.6	6.1
1964	25.2	438.1	401.2	5.8	6.3
1965	27.4	473.2	432.8	5.8	6.3
1966	30.4	511.9	466.3	5.9	6.5
1967	33.6	546.3	492.1	6.2	6.8
1968	37.8	591.0	536.2	6.4	7.0
1969	42.8	634.4	579.5	6.7	7.4
1970	46.8	689.5	616.8	6.8	7.6
1971	50.1	744.4	664.9	6.7	7.5

*Includes expenses for health insurance.
Source: United States Department of Commerce.
By permission of the Health Insurance Institute, 277 Park Avenue, New York, N. Y. 10017.

1966 and 1971. In those same years, the cost of the patient's average stay in the hospital rose 94 percent. The patient stayed in a community hospital an average of 8.0 days. Total operating costs of community hospitals increased from $2 billion in 1950 to $22 billion in 1971 because wages of hospital employees were placed on parity with wages of industrial employees.

How well is the average American prepared to pay for medical and hospital care? A 1972 survey of 273,000 employees with group health insurance revealed the following:

55 percent had basic hospital, surgical, or medical expense coverage.

85 percent had miscellaneous hospital expenses of $300 or more.

99 percent had surgical coverage of maximum benefits of $300 or more.

TABLE 6-3
PERSONAL CONSUMPTION EXPENDITURES FOR
MEDICAL CARE
In the United States
(billions of dollars)

Year	Total medical care*	Hospital services	Physicians' services	Medicines and appliances	Dentists	Net cost of health insurance	All other medical care
1948	$ 7.5	$ 1.6	$ 2.4	$1.9	$0.9	$0.3	$0.4
1950	8.5	2.0	2.6	2.2	1.0	0.3	0.5
1955	12.3	3.1	3.5	3.0	1.5	0.6	0.6
1960	18.6	5.1	5.3	4.4	2.0	0.8	1.0
1961	19.7	5.6	5.5	4.6	2.1	1.0	1.0
1962	21.4	6.1	6.0	4.9	2.3	1.1	1.1
1963	22.8	6.8	6.4	5.1	2.3	1.1	1.2
1964	25.2	7.7	7.1	5.4	2.6	1.2	1.2
1965	27.4	8.3	7.7	5.9	2.8	1.3	1.4
1966	30.4	9.3	8.4	6.7	3.0	1.4	1.6
1967	33.6	10.7	9.3	7.0	3.3	1.6	1.7
1968	36.8	12.3	10.0	7.6	3.5	1.6	1.9
1969	41.6	14.6	11.5	8.2	3.9	1.6	1.9
1970	45.6	17.0	12.4	8.6	4.3	1.4	1.9
1971	50.1	19.4	13.4	8.9	4.7	1.7	2.0

*In some cases the sum of the items does not equal the "Total medical care" shown, due to rounding.
Note: The data exclude private expenditures in federal, state, city and other government hospitals and nursing homes.
Source: United States Department of Commerce.
By permission of the Health Insurance Institute, 277 Park Avenue, New York, N.Y. 10017.

82 percent had medical benefits paying private physicians' fees for in-hospital visits.

78 percent had medical benefits to help pay for out-of-hospital diagnostic X-ray and/or laboratory services.

92 percent had daily hospital room and board benefits of $30 or more.

21 percent had coverage of up to 31 days of hospital confinement and 11 percent had up to 180 days or more.

About one third of the employees in another survey had hospital expense coverage for 365 days or more.[1]

DEVELOPMENT OF HEALTH INSURANCE

The first company to write health insurance in the United States was founded in 1847. Actually, health insurance developed from the public's demand for insurance against the numerous rail and steamboat

TABLE 6-4
CONSUMER PRICE INDICES FOR MEDICAL CARE ITEMS
In the United States (1967 = 100.0)

Year	All medical care items	Physicians' fees	Dentists' fees	Optometric examina- tion and eyeglasses	Hospital room rates	Prescrip- tions and drugs
1947	48.1	51.4	56.9	67.7	22.0	81.8
1950	53.7	55.2	63.9	73.5	28.9	88.5
1955	64.8	65.4	73.0	77.0	41.5	94.7
1960	79.1	77.0	82.1	85.1	56.3	104.5
1961	81.4	79.0	82.5	87.8	60.6	103.3
1962	82.5	81.3	84.7	89.2	64.9	101.7
1963	85.6	83.1	87.1	89.7	69.0	100.8
1964	87.3	85.2	89.4	90.9	72.4	100.5
1965	89.5	88.3	92.2	92.8	76.6	100.2
1966	93.4	93.4	95.2	95.3	84.0	100.5
1967	100.0	100.0	100.0	100.0	100.0	100.0
1968	106.1	105.6	105.5	103.2	113.2	100.2
1969	113.4	112.9	112.9	107.6	127.9	101.3
1970	120.6	121.4	119.4	113.5	143.9	103.6
1971	128.4	129.8	127.0	120.3	160.8	105.4

Source: United States Department of Labor.
By permission of the Health Insurance Institute, 277 Park Avenue, New York, N. Y. 10017.

accidents of the mid-nineteenth century. By 1864 Americans could buy insurance for accidents of every description, and by 1900 at least 47 American companies issued accident insurance. Both accident and health insurance became available through life insurance companies.

In the early days of health insurance, the policyholder received a replacement of income rather than hospital or surgical benefits. Policies replaced income when the policyholder's illness was due to diabetes, typhoid fever, smallpox, diphtheria, typhus fever, scarlet fever, and a few other diseases. There was a seven-day waiting period before the start of the benefit payments. The health insurance policy had an indemnity limited to 26 consecutive weeks.

Rising costs of medical and hospital care in 1929 along with the socioeconomic upheaval at that time made the public aware of the need for a prepayment plan of hospital care. A group of school teachers banded together with Baylor Hospital in Dallas, Texas, to provide themselves with hospital care on a prepayment basis. This was the origin of the Blue Cross service concept of hospital care and had a profound effect on the insurance companies, who began to offer policies to reimburse the holder for hospital and surgical care.

TABLE 6-5
PERCENTAGE DISTRIBUTION OF HEALTH INSURANCE
BENEFIT PAYMENTS BY GEOGRAPHIC REGION
in the United States, 1970

Region	Percentage
New England	6.0
Middle Atlantic	20.0
East North Central	24.0
West North Central	8.0
South Atlantic	12.0
East South Central	5.0
West South Central	6.0
Mountain	3.0
Central Pacific	14.0

Source: Health Insurance Institute, 277 Park Avenue, New York, N.Y. 10017.

Group health insurance became a fringe benefit of collective bargaining when industrial wages were not allowed to be increased during World War II. Three events in the postwar period provided health insurance with its rapid growth. First, the United States Supreme Court permitted fringe benefits, including health insurance, to be legitimate parts of the bargaining process when labor negotiated contracts with management. Second, costs for health care escalated to such an extent that the public needed protection. Third, the continuing improvement of health insurance provided new coverage and more benefits than existing coverages.

Insurance for major medical expenses grew rapidly in the postwar period because it paid for all types of medical expenses—both in and out of a hospital—as prescribed by a physician. Hospital care and special hospital services such as drugs, operating room and anesthesia, surgical procedures and other professional medical care, nursing, diagnostic services, appliances, special medications, and certain types of dental care were included in major medical expense insurance. The health benefits payments for 1970 by geographic region and by type of coverage are listed in Tables 6-5 and 6-6.

Long-term disability income insurance was available after World War II because of the public's need for income during the time of disability and the financial emergencies accompanying the disability. The duration of time for which the disability income benefits have been payable has increased steadily. Many long-term coverages pay benefits for more than two years. Short-term disability benefits may be limited to 26 weeks or continue up to two years.

TABLE 6-6
HEALTH INSURANCE BENEFIT PAYMENTS OF
INSURANCE COMPANIES, BY TYPE OF COVERAGE
In the United States
(000 omitted)

| | 1970 | 1971 | | |
| | | | Under | Age 65 |
Type of coverage	Total	Total	age 65	and over
Total	$9,089,084	$9,497,317	$9,069,393	$427,924
Disability income*	1,816,584	1,774,968	1,686,745	88,223
Hospital expense	3,382,193	3,449,667	3,276,685	172,982
Surgical expense	856,254	878,746	843,457	35,289
Regular medical expense	415,726	430,055	404,773	25,282
Major medical expense	2,478,163	2,788,361	2,684,703	103,658
Dental expense	140,164	175,520	173,030	2,490

*Excludes accidental death and dismemberment benefits of $246,733,000 in 1970 and
$226,920,000 in 1971.
Note: The "Hospital expense," "Surgical expense," and "Regular medical expense"
categories exclude benefits for hospital, surgical and medical expenses for major
medical expense policyholders.
Source: Health Insurance Association of America.

Since World War II, health insurance coverages have grown broader
(Fig. 6-1). Hospitalization benefits have risen from $10 per day to $60
per day or higher. More days of hospitalization per illness are covered.
Allowances for special hospital services have risen from $100 to $500, and
higher. Coverages for surgical care have had comparable increases. With
Medicare in effect, most major medical policies terminate at age 65.
However, some insurance companies provide lifetime coverage on a
guaranteed renewable basis.[2]

HEALTH INSURANCE TERMINOLOGY

Numerous terms appear in a discussion of commercial health insurance. Some terms commonly used are therefore defined.

Allocated benefits. Payments provided in some policies for certain specified hospital
services, such as X rays, to a maximum amount.

Association group. Group insurance provided to a trade or business association by
which all members are protected under one master health insurance contract.

Blanket medical expense. A provision in loss-of-income policies providing payment for hospital and medical expenses to a maximum without limitation on
individual types of medical expenses.

Blanket policy. A health insurance contract that protects all members of a certain
group against a specific hazard.

Blue Cross. An independent, nonprofit membership corporation providing protection against costs of hospital care.

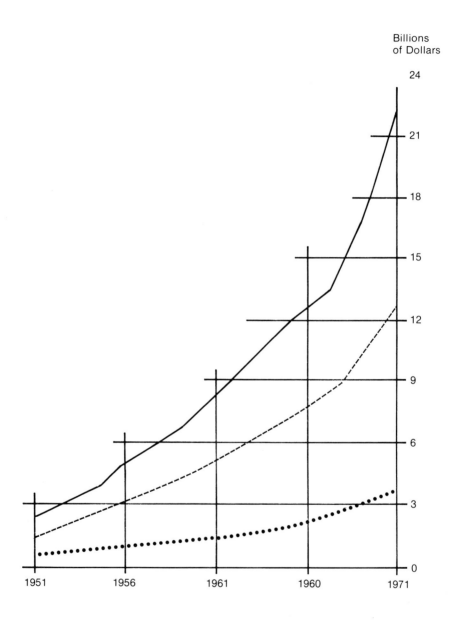

FIGURE 6-1

Distribution of health insurance premiums in the United States, 1951-1971. Insurance company loss-of-income plans, dotted line; insurance company hospital-
medical plans, including surgical, dental, and major medical premiums, broken
line; Blue Cross, Blue Shield, and other hospital medical plans, solid line. (Redrawn
from graph of Health Insurance Institute, 277 Park Avenue, New York, N.Y.
10017.)

Blue Shield. An independent, nonprofit membership corporation providing protection against costs of surgery and other items of medical care.

Coinsurance. A policy provision, frequently found in major medical insurance, by which both the insured person and the insurance company share, in a specified ratio, the hospital and medical expenses resulting from an illness or injury.

Comprehensive major medical insurance. A policy designed to give the protection offered by both a basic and major medical health insurance policy. It is characterized by a low deductible amount, a coinsurance feature, and high maximum benefits, usually $10,000 to $50,000 and more.

Deductible. In major medical insurance plans, that portion of covered hospital and medical charges which an insured person must pay before his policy's benefits begin.

Disability. A physical or mental condition that renders an insured person incapable of performing one or more duties of his regular occupation.

Disability income insurance. A form of health insurance providing periodic payments to replace income when the insured is disabled, temporarily or permanently.

Double indemnity. A policy provision, usually associated with death, that doubles payment of designated benefits when certain kinds of accidents occur.

Elective benefits. A benefit that a policyholder may choose in lieu of the usual compensation payable for certain injuries.

Evidence of insurability. Any statement or proof of a person's physical condition or occupation affecting his acceptance for insurance.

Exclusions. Specific hazards or conditions listed in the policy for which the insurer will not pay benefits.

Family expense policy. A policy that insures both the policyholder and his immediate dependents.

Grace period. A specified time after a policy's premium payment is due in which the policyholder may make such payment and during which the protection of the policy continues.

Guaranteed renewable policy. A policy that the insured has the right to continue in force by the timely payment of premiums to a specified age (such as 60 or 65) or for a lifetime, during which time the insurance company has no right to unilaterally make any change in any provision of the policy while the policy is in force, but may make changes in premium rates by policyholder class.

Health insurance. A generic term applying to all types of insurance indemnifying or reimbursing for costs of hospital and medical care or loss of income arising from an illness or injury. Sometimes, it is called "Accident and Health Insurance" or "Disability Insurance."

Hospital benefits. Benefits provided under a policy for hospital charges incurred by an insured person because of an illness or injury.

Hospital expense insurance. Health insurance protection against the costs of hospital care resulting from the illness or injury of an insured person.

Hospital-medical insurance. A term used to indicate protection that provides benefits toward the cost of any or all of the numerous health care services normally covered under various health insurance plans.

Indemnity. A benefit paid by an insurance company for a loss insured under a policy.

Individual insurance. Policies to provide protection to the policyholder and/or his family (as distinct from group and blanket insurance).

Injury independent of all other means. An injury resulting from an accident, provided that the accident was not caused by an illness.

Insurance clause. The clause that indicates the parties to a health insurance contract, sets forth the type of loss covered, and broadly defines the benefits to be paid.

Lapse. Termination of a policy upon the policyholder's failure to pay the premium within the time required.

Limited policies. Contracts covering only certain diseases or accidents.

Loss-of-income benefits. Payments made to an insured person to help replace income lost through inability to work because of the insured's disability.

Major medical expense insurance. Policies especially designed to help offset the heavy medical expenses resulting from catastrophic or prolonged illness or injury. They provide benefit payments for 75 percent to 80 percent of all types of medical expenses above a deductible amount paid by the insured person. The maximum amount provided by the policy may be $10,000 to $20,000 to $50,000 or more.

Miscellaneous expenses. In connection with hospital insurance, hospital charges other than room and board, such as X-rays, drugs, laboratory fees, and other supplementary charges.

Noncancellable, or noncancellable and guaranteed renewable, policy. A policy that the insured has the right to continue in force to a specified age, such as to age 65, by the timely payment of premiums. During the specified period the insurance company has no right to unilaterally make any change in any provision of the policy while it is in force.

Nonoccupational policy. A contract that insures a person against off-the-job accident or sickness. It does not cover disability resulting from injury or sickness covered by Workmen's Compensation. Group Accident and Sickness policies are frequently nonoccupational.

Partial disability. An illness or injury that prevents an insured person from performing one or more of the functions of his regular job.

Preexisting condition. A physical condition of an insured person that existed prior to the issuance of his policy.

Premium. Periodic payment required to keep a policy in force.

Principal sum. A lump-sum payment made upon the insured person's accidental death.

Probationary period. A specified number of days after the date of the issuance of the policy during which coverage is not afforded for sickness. The purpose of the period is to eliminate benefits for sickness actually contracted before the policy went into force.

Proration. Adjustment of benefits paid because of a mistake in the amount of the premiums paid or the existence of other insurance covering the same accident or disability.

Qualified impairment insurance. A form of substandard or special class insurance that restricts benefits for the insured's particular condition.

Recurring clause. A provision in some health insurance policies that specifies a period of time during which the recurrence of a condition is considered a continuation of a prior period of disability or hospital confinement.

Regular medical expense insurance. Coverage that provides benefits toward the cost of such services as physician's fees for nonsurgical care in the hospital, at home, or in a physician's office and X-rays or laboratory tests performed outside the hospital.

Rider. A legal document that modifies the protection of a policy, either expanding or decreasing its benefits or adding or excluding certain conditions from the policy's coverage.

Risk (impaired or substandard). An insurance applicant whose physical condition does not meet the physical standards for normal health.

Senior citizen policies. Contracts insuring persons 65 years of age or over. In most instances these policies supplement the coverage afforded by Medicare.

Short-term disability income insurance. A provision to pay benefits to a covered disabled person as long as he remains disabled for a specified period not exceeding two years.

Specific disease insurance. A policy that provides benefits, usually of large amounts, toward the expense of the treatment of the disease or diseases named in the policy.

Substandard health insurance. An individual policy issued to a person who cannot meet the normal health requirements of a standard health insurance policy. Protection is given in consideration of an increase in premium, through a waiver of medical condition, or under a special qualified impairment policy.

Surgical expense insurance. Health insurance policies that provide benefits toward the surgeon's fees. Benefits usually consist of scheduled amounts for each surgical procedure.

Surgical schedule. A list of cash allowances that are payable for various types of operations, with the maximum amounts based upon the severity of the operations.

Time Limit. The period of time in which a notice of claim or proof of a loss must be filed.

Total disability. An illness or injury that prevents an insured person from continuously performing every duty pertaining to his occupation or from engaging in any other type of work for renumeration. (This definition varies among insurance companies.)

Unallocated benefit. A policy provision that provides reimbursement to a maximum amount for the costs of all extra miscellaneous hospital services but does not specify how much will be paid for each type of service.

Waiting period. The duration of time between the beginning of an insured person's disability and the start of the policy's benefits.

Waiver. An agreement attached to a policy that exempts from coverage certain disabilities or injuries normally covered by the policy.

Waiver of premium. A provision included in some policies to exempt the insured person from paying premiums while he is disabled during the life of the contract.

Written premium. The entire amount of premiums on all policies issued by an insurance company in a year.[3]

SOURCES AND GENERAL TYPES OF
HEALTH INSURANCE

Private organizations offering health insurance may be insurance companies and nonprofit groups. Insurance companies may be the mutual type (member pool) or the stock company type. There are more than 1045 commercial insurance companies. Examples of nonprofit groups are labor unions, industrially sponsored groups, credit unions, Blue Cross and/or Blue Shield, and fraternal groups. A second source of health insurance is the federal government.

Medicare

Title 18, Medicare, Social Security Act, became effective July 1, 1966, for persons age 65 and over. Medicare consists of two parts. Part A is a basic compulsory program of hospital insurance. Part B is medical insurance to help pay physicians' fees for persons entitled to Part A—hospital insurance. Part A is financed by special contributions from employees and self-employed persons, with employers paying an equal amount. Part B is financed by monthly premiums paid by the enrollee and by a specified amount paid by the federal government. The Social Security Administration is responsible for the administration of Title 18.

The general benefits under Title 18 will be discussed. Readers should be aware that lengths of time, costs to the subscriber, amounts paid by Medicare, services to the subscriber, and other Medicare items may be changed with each Congressional action. Current regulations may be obtained from the local Social Security Administration office.

The hospital insurance (Part A) provides three kinds of hospital and posthospital benefits. It covers a bed patient in a hospital, a bed patient in an extended care facility, or a patient at home receiving home health services. In Medicare, the term *benefit period* is often used. A benefit period is a period of time for measuring use of hospital insurance benefits. The period begins when the Medicare recipient enters the hospital. It ends when the patient has not been a bed patient in a hospital or nursing home for 60 days in a row. A new benefit period begins the next time the person enters a hospital or nursing home. There is no limit to the number of benefit periods a person may have.

Bed patient care for a stated number of days may be in a participating general care, tuberculosis, or psychiatric hospital if these facilities meet standards of high quality health care, do not charge the Medicare beneficiary for services paid by Medicare, and do not discriminate on basis of race, color, or national origin. Payment covers services for 90 days. Each person has a "lifetime reserve" of 60 additional days. Care in a psychiatric hospital has a lifetime benefit limit of 190 days. The bed patient benefits include these services:

Bed in a semiprivate room and all meals, including special diets.

Operating room charges.

Regular nursing services (intensive care nursing included).

Drugs furnished by the hospital.

Laboratory tests.

X-ray and other radiology services.

Medical supplies such as splints and casts.

Use of appliances and equipment furnished by the hospital such as a wheelchair, crutches, and braces.

Medical social services.

Hospital insurance can help pay for inpatient care in a Canadian hospital if the subscriber becomes ill or injured while traveling through Canada between Alaska and another state.

A hospital patient may recover to the point that he does not require intensive care at a hospital but needs full-time skilled nursing and other health services that cannot be provided in his home. This patient may be transferred to an extended care facility (nursing home or rehabilitative facility). All covered services in an approved extended care facility are paid for the first 20 days in each benefit period. Medicare also pays the partial cost for 80 more days in that same benefit period. To qualify for extended care benefits, a patient must have been in a hospital for three days prior to being transferred to the extended care facility by his physician. Also, the patient must enter the extended care facility within 14 days of leaving the hospital. The following services are included in extended care benefits after leaving the hospital:

Bed in a semiprivate room and all meals, including special diets.

Regular nursing services.

Drugs furnished by the extended care or skilled nursing facility.

Physical, occupational, and speech therapy.

Medical supplies such as splints and casts.

Use of appliances and equipment furnished by the facility such as a wheelchair, crutches, and braces.

Medical social services.

Home Health benefits are given to the patient who has been in the hospital for at least three days (or has been in an extended care facility *after* being a hospital patient for at least three days). If the patient then requires nurses' or technicians' services that can be provided at home, the physician may set up a schedule of treatments and permit the patient to go home. Medicare hospital insurance will pay for 100 home health visits a year after the start of one benefit period and before the start of another. The patient must be receiving treatment for the same condition which required his admission to a hospital in the first place. The patient must be confined to his home. The physician must determine that the patient needs home health care and establish a home health plan for the patient within 14 days after the patient's discharge from a hospital or an extended care facility. These services are included:

Part-time skilled nursing care, physical or speech therapy.

Occupational therapy.

Part-time services of home health aides.

Medical social services.

Medical supplies and appliances furnished by the agency.

Since January 1, 1973, Medicare has helped to pay for covered in-patient care in a foreign hospital if the qualified foreign hospital is closer than a United States hospital.

The medical insurance under Part B of Medicare automatically covers persons who were entitled to hospital insurance in July 1973 or later unless those persons say they do not want the medical insurance. Medical insurance helps to pay physicians' fees, limited dental services, outpatient hospital services, radiology and pathology services when in a hospital, home health benefits, other medical services and supplies, ambulance services, outpatient physical therapy and speech pathology services, and emergency outpatient care from certain nonparticipating hospitals. The insured makes a monthly payment, and the federal government pays that same amount or more. After the patient's bills for covered services go over a specified sum each year, the medical insurance pays 80 percent of the reasonable charges for the remaining part of that year. Some of physicians' services are:

Medical and surgical services by a doctor of medicine or osteopathy.

Certain medical and surgical services by a doctor of dental medicine or a doctor of dental surgery.

Certain services by podiatrists which they are legally authorized to perform by the state in which they practice.

Other services that are ordinarily furnished in the physician's office and included in his bill such as diagnostic tests and procedures, medical supplies, services of his office nurse, drugs and biologicals which cannot be self-administered, and limited services by chiropractors.

Payment can be made no matter where the patient is treated: hospital, physician's office, extended care facility, patient's home, or group practice or other clinic. The patient selects his physician.

Outpatient hospital services are given to persons going to the hospital for diagnosis or treatment but who are not admitted as patients in the hospital. Some of the outpatient hospital benefits are:

Laboratory services.

X-ray and other radiology services.

Emergency room services and outpatient clinic services.

Medical supplies such as splints and casts.

Other diagnostic services.

The same kind of home health benefits covered under hospital insurance are available. The person does not have to be hospitalized first to get home health benefits under medical insurance. The person can have 100 home health visits each year. The home health benefits are:
Part-time nursing care, physical therapy or speech therapy.
Occupational therapy.
Part-time services of home health aides.
Medical social services.
Medical supplies and appliances furnished by the agency.
The agency making the home visits will bill the patient for any part of the specified amount deductible not met by the patient.

Other medical services and supplies necessary in the treatment of an illness or injury and provided in medical insurance are:
Diagnostic laboratory tests furnished by approved independent laboratories.
Radiation therapy and diagnostic X-ray services.
Portable diagnostic X-ray services furnished in the patient's home under a physician's supervision.
Surgical dressings, splints, casts, and similar devices.
Rental or purchase of durable medical equipment such as a wheelchair prescribed by a physician for use in the patient's home.
Devices (other than dental) to replace all or part of an internal body organ. This includes corrective lenses after a cataract operation and certain colostomy equipment and supplies.
Certain ambulance services.

Outpatient physical therapy and speech pathology services are covered by medical insurance when they are under the direct supervision of a physician or when they are provided for as part of home health services. These physical therapy and speech pathology services may be provided by the hospital, extended care facility, home health agency, clinic, rehabilitative agency, or public health agency if established and periodically reviewed by a physician. Since July 1, 1973, home and office services furnished by a licensed physical therapist have been covered under medical insurance.

Emergency outpatient care from certain nonparticipating hospitals is covered under the medical insurance. The hospital may bill Medicare for its share of the charges. The hospital may bill the patient for the amount deductible plus a specified percentage of the remaining reasonable charges. If the hospital bills the patient for the entire amount, the medical insurance of Medicare pays 80 percent of the reasonable charges above the specified deductible amount.

Limited coverage of dental services in the medical insurance includes only services involving surgery of the jaw or related structures or setting of fractures of the jaw or facial bones.

Radiology and pathology services are included. When the subscriber is a bed patient in a hospital, these services are paid 100 percent by medical insurance. The hospital must be a participating or otherwise qualified hospital for receiving Medicare funds.

Ambulance services include ambulance transportation by an approved ambulance service to a hospital or extended care facility. The ambulance service must meet Medicare requirements as to the ambulance itself, equipment, and personnel. Also, the ambulance service must be required because other types of transportation might endanger the patient's health. When the patient is taken to a facility other than the nearest one that can provide appropriate care, only the reasonable charges for ambulance transportation to the nearest facility can be allowed. Medical insurance can help pay for ambulance services from one hospital to another, from a hospital to an extended care facility, or from a hospital or extended care facility to the patient's home.

After January 1, 1973, Medicare extended its coverage to help pay for medically necessary physicians' services and ambulance services in connection with hospitalization when the subscriber is in a foreign hospital. The subscriber must live in a border area of the United States and a qualified foreign hospital must be closer to him than a United States hospital.

Instructions are given to the subscriber if he becomes a patient in a hospital which does not take part in Medicare. These include how the patient can claim medical insurance benefits, when the first medical insurance claim is sent to Medicare, and what procedures to take if the subscriber belongs to a group practice prepayment plan.[4]

Medicaid

A companion measure to Medicare and a medical assistance program—Medicaid (Title 19)—became effective January 1, 1966. This federal-state program of medical assistance for the needy has received a lot of attention because all levels of government are involved. Medicaid is financed by state and federal funds. Federal funds vary from 50 to 83 percent inversely in relation to a state's per capita income.

Medicaid coverage varies from state to state. It includes services by physicians, dentists, pharmacists, optometrists, podiatrists, chiropractors, hospitals, extended care facilities, and home health services. Medicaid includes preventive, diagnostic, therapeutic, and rehabilitative services. Medicaid provides higher payments and consolidates the separate programs of medical assistance found in Old Age Assistance, Aid for Dependent Children, Aid to the Blind, and Aid to the Permanently and Totally Dependent. It also extends medical assistance to persons who have sufficient financial resources to take care of day-to-day expenses, but who cannot afford to pay for medical care.

A state, to qualify its Medicaid program under Title 19, must submit an acceptable plan to the Department of Health, Education, and Welfare. The plan must include inpatient hospital services, outpatient hospital services, laboratory and X-ray services, extended care services, and physicians' services. Each state, with federal approval, establishes the amounts of income and resources an applicant may have and still be eligible for benefits. Usually, all persons on welfare and public assistance are eligible.

By July, 1977, all states must furnish comprehensive care and services to all needy and medically needy of not only the minimum five required services to enter the program but also fifteen other services. The reader should be aware that all stated lengths of time, services to persons receiving assistance, and other items in Medicaid may be changed with each Congressional action.

Other Governmental Health Insurance

In addition to Medicare and Medicaid, the social security program provides disability benefits and supplemental security income to persons in financial need. Protection against the loss of earnings because of disability became effective in 1954. The Social Security Amendments of 1972 provide for the following protection:

1. The waiting period for disability benefits was reduced to five months.
2. Certain persons disabled before age 22 can receive disability benefits.
3. More blind workers are eligible for disability than previously.
4. Cash disability benefits are available to survivors of disabled workers who died prior to filing for disability benefits in the social security program.
5. Medicare protection is provided to persons under 65 who have been entitled to Social Security disability benefits for two or more years.
6. Cash benefits can be given to disabled widows, disabled dependent widowers, and disabled surviving divorced wives of workers who were insured at death. The disabled surviving divorced wives have to comply with certain stipulations. Benefits are payable as early as age 50.

A disabled person, not 22 years of age, can get cash Social Security disability benefits on the earnings of a parent.

A person whose vision is no better than 20/200 even with glasses or who has a limited visual field of 20 degrees or less is blind under Social Security regulations. If not working, the blind person can receive monthly benefits. If the blind person is working, he may be able to have his rights to future benefits protected under other special provisions in the law for blind people.

A disabled worker under 62 years of age and entitled to both Social Security disability benefits and workmen's compensation can receive payments to the worker and his family not exceeding 80 percent of his average monthly earnings before he became disabled. Medical evidence is asked to support any claim for Social Security disability benefits. This evidence may come from the physician, hospital, clinic, or institution where the disabled has been treated. If the disabled worker is asked to have medical examinations and tests to establish his disability, the federal government pays these expenses. Decision of disability is made by the vocational rehabilitation agency in the state where the disabled worker lives.

Supplemental security income in the form of monthly cash benefits became available in January, 1974, to persons in financial need who are 65 or older or blind or disabled. This program replaces federal-state programs of public assistance payments to people who are 65 or older or blind or disabled.

In addition to the supplemental income, eligible persons may have a small income, but they must have little or no cash income and not own much real or personal property such as stocks, jewelry, or other valuables that can be turned into cash. This supplemental security income is not the same as Social Security.

All stated lengths of time, services to persons receiving assistance, and other items in other governmental health insurance plans may be changed by Congressional action. The reader should secure the most recent regulations.

GROUP HEALTH INSURANCE

Group health insurance represents more than 72 percent of all health insurance premiums paid to commercial insurance companies in the United States. The group is underwritten as an individual. The insurance company or nonprofit group provides facilities to administer the group plan. Accurate and valid records of employee eligibility are kept by the insurance company or nonprofit group so that benefits meet the needs of the individuals in the group, beneficiaries receive correct funds, and premiums are collected. Most group health insurance is written without the employee undergoing a medical examination. The trend in group health insurance has been for the employer to bear the whole cost. Some advantages are that the amount for health insurance becomes tax deductible, provides a fringe benefit for employees, promotes the health of employees, and permits the employer full control over the plan. Workmen's compensation provided by state laws is group insurance. Employers are responsible for providing workmen's compensation. When group health insurance is not paid by the employer, the advantages for the participant are that (1) premiums are less expensive than individual premiums, (2) broader coverage is provided, and (3) shorter waiting periods are available before benefits become effective. Disadvantages of group insurance are that the benefits of the insurance are limited to the basic needs of the majority within the group. Benefits apply only so long as the employee remains on the job. Employees retiring after being members of the group for a given length of time may not continue to be members of the group health insurance plan. More and more, employees are being given the right to convert to standard health insurance plans to prevent loss of protection when they leave the group.

Several specific types of group health insurance will be presented in the following pages: (1) hospital expense insurance; (2) surgical expense insurance; (3) regular medical expense insurance; (4) major medical expense insurance; (5) loss of income protection; (6) dental expense insurance; and (7) various plans such as the Healthcare Program, Ameriplan, Health Security Act, Kaiser-Permanente Medical Care Program, Medicredit Plan, National Health Insurance Standards Act, and Health Maintenance Organization Act.

Hospital Expense Insurance

More than 180 million Americans have hospital expense insurance (Fig. 6-2). These plans cover the partial cost of hospital room and board for a stated length of time. Meals and special diets, general nursing services, X-ray examinations, all drugs and medicines, laboratory examinations, use of the operating room and the cystoscopic room, oxygen and oxygen therapy, anesthetic materials and services, electrocardio-

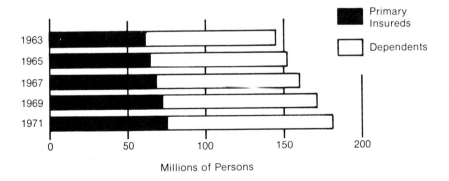

FIGURE 6-2

Number of primary insurers and dependents protected by hospital expense insurance issued by all insurers in the United States. (By permission of the Health Insurance Institute, 277 Park Avenue, New York, N. Y. 10017)

grams, physiotherapy and hydrotherapy, radiation therapy, and blood transfusion service are usually included. The plan designates a specific dollar amount limitation for room and board on a daily basis. Maximum dollar amounts for other expenses incurred are stated in the plan. There is a limit on the number of days of hospitalization. Most plans exclude long-lasting health conditions such as cancer or mental illness. Payment by the insuring company or nonprofit group is accomplished by either cash benefits to the insured or payment of services directly to the hospital. In the cash benefits to the insured, the insuring company or nonprofit group reimburses the insured for most of the hospital expenses. When the payment of services goes directly to the hospital, the patient and family are not burdened with transferring the insurance benefits to the hospital. Before subscribing to any hospital expense insurance, the subscriber should be familiar with the services offered by the plan.

Insurance companies protect over 113 million Americans, or 63 percent of the total number, with hospital expense insurance. Blue Cross and/or medical society-approved plans cover at least 78 million or 43 percent of the total number with hospital expense insurance. Independent plans, such as those with labor unions, protect 9 million or 5 percent of the total number with hospital expense insurance. These numbers of persons exceed 100 percent because many persons have coverage through more than one type of insuring source.

Surgical Expense Insurance

At least 165 million Americans have surgical expense insurance. These plans cover the partial cost of the physicians' services. There are schedules which state the amount of money allotted toward defraying costs for surgery of the abdomen; amputations; surgical repair of dislocations and fractures; surgery of the eyes, ears, nose and throat; general surgery such as treatment for varicose veins and thyroidectomy; gynecologic procedures such as hysterectomy; neurosurgery; and surgery involving many other specialized branches of medicine.

Surgical expense insurance can be sold as a separate form of insurance but usually is jointly offered with the hospital expense plan. The schedule of benefits paid to the subscriber or to the physician includes the maximum amounts paid by the insurance on each type of surgery. Coverage usually includes both preoperative and postoperative care. Most physicians have agreed to accept payment under these surgical expense insurance plans unless the patient has substantial income.

Insurance companies protect over 102 million persons, or 62 percent of the total number of persons covered by surgical expense insurance. Blue Cross-Blue Shield protect more than 69 million, or 42 percent of the total. Independent plans insure 11 million persons, or 7 percent of the total number of persons covered. These numbers of persons exceed

100 percent because many persons have coverage through more than one type of insuring source.

From 1961 to 1971, the total number of persons with surgical expense protection from insurance companies increased 37 percent (Fig. 6-3). The number of persons protected through Blue Cross-Blue Shield and medical society-approved plans increased by 38 percent. The number of persons subscribing to surgical expense insurance under independent plans increased 35 percent.

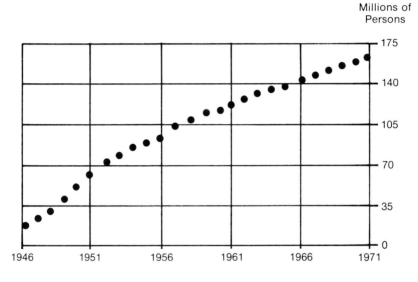

Millions of Persons

FIGURE 6-3

Number of persons with surgical expense protection in the United States. (By permission of the Health Insurance Institute, 277 Park Avenue, New York, N. Y. 10017)

Regular Medical Insurance

Regular medical insurance pays for the physician's services other than surgical fees. It provides predetermined amounts for physician's visits with the patient in a hospital, in his home, or at the physician's office. Some regular medical insurance plans also provide payments for diagnostic X-ray and laboratory expenses. Usually the subscriber must have hospital expense insurance and surgical expense insurance, either separately or in combination, in order to purchase regular medical insurance.

At least 144 million Americans have regular medical insurance. More than 79.5 million persons, or 55 percent, have regular medical insurance from insurance companies. Blue Cross-Blue Shield and medical society-approved regular medical insurance plans protect 65 million persons, or 45 percent of the total. Independent plans of regular medical insurance protect 11 million persons, or 8 percent. These numbers of persons exceed 100 percent because many persons have coverage through more than one type of insuring source. From 1961 to 1971, the number of Americans with regular medical expense insurance increased 82 percent.

Major Medical Expense Insurance

Major medical expense insurance helps pay for virtually all types of medical expense—both in and out of a hospital—as prescribed by a physician. It includes hospital care and special hospital services such as drugs, operating room, and anesthesia; surgery and other medical care; skilled nursing services; special medications; diagnostic services; appliances; and certain types of dental care. Coverage for nursing home care, ambulatory psychiatric care, and other health needs of the subscriber is available. Sometimes, labeled as "catastrophic" medical expense insurance, this type of insurance protects the subscriber against serious and/or prolonged illnesses.

Some of the distinguishing features of major medical insurance are the large dollar amounts for the benefits ($5,000 to $50,000, for one illness or one policy year) and the large deductible amounts paid by the policyholder. The policyholder pays a certain amount or percentage of the medical expense before the insurer will accept the claim for the balance. The claim is applied to one person unless the family of the policyholder is included in the policy.

At least 81 million Americans have major medical expense insurance. This type of health insurance is growing rapidly. Some plans include eye examinations and eyeglasses. Often the major medical expense insurance is provided as a supplement to basic hospital-surgical expense insurance plans or regular medical insurance plans. Of the 81 million Americans with major medical expense insurance, insurance companies protect 75 million with group policies and 6 million with individual and family policies. Of the 75 million, supplementary plans were held by 55.5 million persons and comprehensive plans by 19.5 million persons. Comprehensive plans might include hospital expense, surgical expense, regular medical expense, and major medical expense insurance in one coverage.

Loss of Income Protection

Often called "disability income insurance," loss of income protection is designed to provide the policyholder or wage earner with regular weekly or monthly cash payments in the event that wages are discontinued as a result of illness or accident. This coverage may be in the form of short-term protection—maximum benefit periods of two years. Long-term protection may have benefit periods beyond two years.

Loss of income protection may be called "accident insurance," which covers death or dismemberment of an insured individual due to an accident. Payments for loss of life, a hand, a foot, an eye, speech, and hearing are typical benefits. These plans have no coverage for suicide or self-inflicted injury, bodily or mental infirmity or disease, or medical or surgical treatment not connected with an accident.

Loss of income protection may be long-term disability insurance. This insurance supplements ordinary disability insurance and guarantees 60 to 70 percent of the subscriber's monthly income at the time of the disability. Usually it is sold in multiples of $100, has waiting periods imposed before the policyholder may make a claim, and is separate insurance. At least 12 million persons are covered by long-term disability policies of insurance companies.

More than 59 million Americans are covered by short-term loss of income protection through insurance companies or other plans. At least 41 million workers have short-term disability income policies from insurance companies. Of these 41 million, group policies were held by 32 million workers and individual plans were subscribed by 12 million. More than 16.5 million American policyholders subscribe to short-term loss of income protection through formal paid sick leave plans of private industries and of civilian government. Many persons have both long-term and short-term coverages.

Dental Expense Insurance

Dental expense insurance is similar to medical expense insurance. It helps pay for normal dental expense as well as damage caused by accidents and is usually available through insurance company group plans, prepayment plans, and dental service cooperations.

The American Dental Association recognizes three types of dental prepayment coverage. First, there are dental service corporations organized by state dental societies on a nonprofit basis. These corporations are legally constituted to negotiate and administer contracts for group dental care. In addition, the patient has his choice of dentists. Second, there are commercial insurance companies offering dental prepayment coverage. In this coverage the patient is also allowed to choose his dentist. Third, dentists working in a clinic either full or part-time may provide prepayment plans. The patient does not select his dentist.

At least 7.8 million persons have some dental insurance coverage from insurance companies. More than $175.5 million have been paid by them as benefits in a single year. Persons age 65 and over received more than $2.5 million while persons under 65 years received the rest. All sources of dental insurance benefits in one year may amount to $250.5 million.

A recent study of group practice using capitation payment and a service corporation system using fee-for-services and a table of allowances compared utilization rates for one or more dental visits, prophylaxes, extractions, crown and bridge units, root canal therapy, partial dentures and full dentures. Group practice had a higher number of dental visits, prophylaxis rates, and removable prosthetic rates. Group practice and open panel (service corporation system) had the same extraction rates and crown and bridge rates.[5]

The Healthcare Program

Following two years of study and consultation with medical economists and other health experts, the Health Insurance Association of America offered an insurance proposal, the Healthcare Program. The Program is designed to correct problems in the organization, delivery, and financing of personal health services for the entire population. The Health Insurance Association of America represents more than 300 insurance companies which issue approximately 80 percent of the health insurance written by the insurance companies in the United States. The program consists of six parts.

Part I is designed to increase the supply of physicians, nurses, and other health personnel. Recommendations are made for expansion of federal grants and loan programs to help students pay for their medical educations. Also, there are recommendations that parts of the loans made to student doctors, dentists, and other health personnel be cancelled for each year that the graduate agrees to serve in a community having severe shortages of such personnel.

Part II is aimed at keeping persons out of the hospital. Special emphasis in the Healthcare Program would be placed on preventive care benefits and ambulatory health care centers. Such health services as diagnosis, treatment, rehabilitation, mental health services, dental care, drugs, care of vision, family planning, immunization against diseases, and health education would be provided in the ambulatory health care centers.

Part III is designed to reduce duplication of expensive hospital and health facilities by improvement of local health planning agencies. This part of the Healthcare Program contains provisions to give local health planning agencies more control over organizing health facilities in their communities.

Part IV is designed to reduce rising health costs to the American family while improving the quality of care. Standard accounting systems and upgrading the efficiency of manpower in hospitals are two recommendations. Also, it proposes an active committee of physicians to constantly check the care each patient receives in a hospital. Unnecessary operations, overly long hospital stays, and unneeded treatment would be curbed.

Part V recommends a full-time Council of Health Policy Advisers to the President which would establish national health goals. This Council would be in one of the highest levels of government and would give health top priority with other national priorities.

Part VI would provide for delivering the full potential of American medicine to as many persons as possible in the shortest time. The Healthcare Program recommends that the federal government establish standards of health insurance benefits to be met by all insurance plans. Regardless of income, all persons would have available these health insurance benefits.

Federally established benefits would be encouraged in existing health insurance plans by tax incentives for employers who include these benefits in their employees' group plans. Persons with individually owned policies would receive similar incentives.[6]

Similar to the American Medical Association's Medicredit plan, the Healthcare Program would cover physicians' services wherever rendered; 12 days of hospital care for each illness, either as inpatient or as an outpatient; dental services; prescribed drugs; prosthetic devices; pregnancy costs; health services at an extended care facility or in the home; and part of the costs of a catastrophic illness. If an employer and a worker share the costs of the insurance, each can deduct for income tax purposes the amount he paid. Low-income persons presently eligible for Medicaid would have the health insurance paid by federal and state funds.

Ameriplan

The American Hospital Association has prepared a health insurance plan, Ameriplan. Three packages of insurance are proposed. One provides standard benefits resembling those of Medicare with additional coverage for such items as maternity and child care. Another package would provide health-maintenance care including annual medical examinations and other laboratory examinations, if ordered by a physician; immunizations; and dental services for children. The third package would protect against costs of a catastrophic illness. To get the health-maintenance and catastrophic illness benefits, a person would first have to subscribe to a private health insurance plan offering standard benefits. Also, the person would have to enroll in a "health corporation" that would not only set standards for health care but also direct funds into educating health personnel and improving such facilities as hospitals.

The aged and low income or poor person now covered by Medicaid would be insured for all three packages of benefits at public expense, with costs paid by the federal government out of general revenues. People who could afford to buy standard health insurance would do so in the same way as they do already. They could enroll in a health corporation and buy health maintenance and catastrophic illness packages. They would not be compelled to buy any insurance packages. Medicare and Medicaid would be ended.

Each state would have a State Health Commission, under the guidance of a National Health Commission. Each state Commission would set payments for care at local levels. The National Commission would establish the range of benefits and standards of quality.

Health Security Act

Sponsored by organized labor, the Health Security Act would include everyone from cradle to the grave. Some $30 billion would be rechanneled from private health insurance programs into the Health Security Act. Each taxpayer would pay through the federal government. There would be no direct charge to patients. Costs would be financed half from general revenues and half from Social Security payroll taxes.

All physicians' fees, hospital charges, 120 days in a skilled-nursing home, prescribed drugs, limited psychiatric care, dental care for children under 15 at the start of this program, and dental care for all persons to age 25 would be paid. The federal government would operate the Health Security Act through a Health Security Board, which would establish standard charges and prepay the bills. Professional panels would check performance of physicians, hospitals, and other health personnel. It is hoped the Health Security Act would stimulate group-practice arrangements.

Kaiser-Permanente Medical Care Program

In 1933 a plan of medical care was offered to 5000 workers building an aqueduct across the California desert. The plan cost ten cents a day for each worker. One of the contractors for the aqueduct was Henry J. Kaiser. He was so pleased with the medical care given to the workers that he offered the plan to other workers at Kaiser's steel mills and shipyards. At the end of World War II, Kaiser opened the medical care plan to the public.

More than 2.3 million persons are members of the Kaiser-Permanente Medical Care Program. At least 2600 physicians, 14,500 nurses, 20,000 other management and health personnel, 23 hospitals, and 58 outpatient medical centers are participating in this plan.

Run on "hard-nosed" business principles, the Kaiser-Permanente program is totally self-supporting. Kaiser hospital administrators strive to keep costs under intelligent control without diminishing quality of care. Hospitals are highly mechanized, relieving nurses of many chores. Expensive kitchens do not have to be maintained because caterers provide precooked, tasty, frozen meals which are heated at the nurse stations. Centralized purchasing helps cut costs. Laboratories serve half a dozen or more hospitals with courier pickup and delivery. A radiation center is available with an apartment house where patients can stay at no cost during treatment.

The purpose of the Kaiser-Permanente Medical Care Program is to organize medical services for the public on a prepayment basis at costs that families with average incomes can afford. It operates on a non-profit basis. The Kaiser plan provides members and their families with complete medical service in the physician's office, in the subscriber's home, or in a hospital, including laboratory examinations and X-rays, at a relatively low cost. Individuals and organized groups may join on a pre-payment basis. The subscriber selects a family physician from the medical staff and has access to all types of medical specialists.

Medicredit Plan

The health insurance plan proposed by the American Medical Association is called Medicredit because it includes income tax credits for costs of private health insurance. Everyone would be eligible except persons over 65 years of age who would be covered by Medicare. Participation in the Medicredit plan would be voluntary.

Persons would buy their own private health insurance. Those who brought health insurance covering 60 days of hospital care, unlimited visits to physicians, and dental surgery would get income tax credits for all or part of their insurance costs, with the amount of credit varying according to the amount of tax owed. A person paying more than $890 in income tax would get credit for only 10 percent of his health insurance costs. Larger credits would be given to people paying less in taxes. Those persons owing no income tax would get from the government free certificates to be used to pay for health insurance. These certificates would replace the existing Medicaid benefits. For the aged, Medicare would be continued. The agencies providing health care would be able to operate freely, without government controls. Subscribers would continue to have full freedom to choose their own physicians and each person would have insurance to cover his family's health needs.

National Health Insurance Standards Act

The National Health Insurance Standards Act would require employers to provide health insurance for their employees who would share in underwriting the cost. Employers would pay 65 percent of the insurance cost for the first two and one half years and a minimum of 75 percent thereafter.

The insurance would cover hospital services, treatment by physicians in and out of hospitals, maternity care, immunizations and other routine safeguards for babies, laboratory fees, and other expenses that are not paid under many health insurance plans now available to subscribers. Also, there would be at least $50,000 in protection against catastrophic illnesses for each member of the employee's family.

The Act would encourage private insurance companies to offer health insurance plans. However, these private companies would be regulated by the federal government to make sure they offer the benefits they claim to offer and at reasonable rates. For persons self-employed and special groups, the states would be required to provide coverage at group rates.

Included in the National Health Insurance Standards Act is the Family Health Insurance Plan. This plan meets the needs of low-income families who would not be covered by the National Health Insurance Standards Act. It would assist families headed by an unemployed person or by a self-employed person whose income was below a specified amount. The Family Health Insurance Plan would replace Medicaid which would be available only to the aged poor, blind, disabled, and some children.

As a part of the Standards Act, there would be health maintenances organizations (HMO's) similar to private group plans now in effect. It is hoped that the HMO would bring together into a single organization the physician, hospital, laboratory and clinic, so that patients could get the right type of medical and hospital care at the right moment. HMO would contract to provide comprehensive care for a fixed annual sum that is determined in advance. HMO would strive to keep members well, prevent them from becoming ill, and treat them as quickly as possible. The HMO would be coupled with the basic insurance plan.

Families could continue to have physicians who practice independently and bill their patients in the traditional way. However, group medical practice would be encouraged to expand so that more persons would have the choice of medical care.

Health Maintenance Organization Act

In the last days of 1973, President Nixon signed a new law to stimulate the spread of Health Maintenance Organizations. More than 5.5 million Americans participate in at least 125 HMO's in operation. It is predicted that by 1978 at least 525 HMO's will be operating with as many as 20 million American subscribers.

HMO is an organization which guarantees to provide basic medical services, whether routine or emergency, to a group of subscribers in a given area for a fixed fee, paid in advance, for a period of a year. The basic services during 24 hours, each day, include

1. Physicians' services, both consultations and referrals to other physicians if necessary.
2. Inpatient and outpatient hospital services, including laboratory, anesthesia, and radiation fees.
3. Emergency care.
4. Health care at home.
5. Medical treatment for alcoholism and narcotic addiction or drug abuse.

6. Short-term psychiatric care.
7. Complete annual medical examinations.
8. Dental examinations and care for children under 12 years of age, including cleaning of teeth and application of fluorides and sealants, if necessary.

Fees for subscribers would vary from one area of the United States to another. HMO physicians emphasize preventive care and treatment.

Some of the advantages of HMO's are medical care under a single roof, one telephone number, 24 hours a day, seven days a week, if no hospitalization is needed. The subscriber will have medical care when he needs it, will not have to fill out complicated forms, will not need to furnish proof of ability to pay, and will not have to have a medical examination when he sees a new physician. Also, one of the physicians will make a house call if the subscriber cannot get to the HMO. The subscriber must have yearly medical examinations and necessary laboratory tests.

Many present HMO contracts do not include dental care, glasses, or prescription drugs. The subscriber pays extra for these services. The subscriber receives the medical or dental care depending on the HMO contract.

The federal government will provide at $325 million until July 1, 1978, to help develop new HMO's and expand existing ones. The funds are in the form of grants, contracts, and loans or loan guarantees. The law encourages creation of new HMO's in rural and inner city populations. Also, the law encourages different HMO's in different situations so as to see how they work, or why they do not work. One third of the policy-making group in an HMO must be people who use the service.

MAIL-ORDER HEALTH INSURANCE

There are at least 170 companies in the mail-order health insurance business in the United States. In 1971, these companies received 2 percent of the total health insurance dollar. Advertising provides the success of these companies' sales which have created enormous problems for state insurance departments. Key complaints are that purchasers are not receiving what the advertisements led them to believe. The advertisements mix fear and greed. One advertisement read, "Get up to $33.33 per day extra cash, in addition to doctor and hospital costs, to spend any way you want." Investigations of the claims made in numerous advertisements showed that only 0.9 percent of the claim payments exceed $500. Also, the Internal Revenue Service has not accepted the premiums of mail-order health insurance as tax deductible, while premiums for medical and basic hospital health insurance of Blue Cross are tax deductible.

Mail-order health insurance plans emphasize monthly benefits to the policyholder when he is hospitalized for an accident or illness. The prevalent, accepted benefit is a daily, not monthly benefit. These mail-order policies indicate that the policyholder must spend a full month in a hospital to get the monthly benefit. The average hospital stay is eight days.

Among the mail-order health insurance plans, there are policy variations such as those policies that cannot be renewed after age 65. Others can be cancelled statewide, and others can be cancelled individually at the company's option. Some companies will not pay claims resulting from ailments a person had when he purchased the policy—usually for two years after policy issuance. Unfortunately five out of every nine persons having mail-order health insurance also have Medicare. Many elderly persons do not know that they have preexisting ailments. Most complaints relate to rejection by the mail-order company to pay benefits because of preexisting ailments. In some mail-order insurance companies the policyholder's childhood is investigated to find a long forgotten ailment. Also, the policy may state that an ailment must have been "medically advised" during the year prior to the policy issuance. This means that if the policyholder has not seen his physician that year, the insurance company reserves the right to rule that the ailment would have been detected if there had been a visit to the physician.

In mail-order health insurance, waiting periods ranging from three to eight days are the rule. Since the average hospital stay is eight days, the mail-order health insurance may pay for that last day only when the policy is an eight-day policy. Many mail-order insurance policies pay nothing for treatment in nursing, convalescent, rehabilitation or extended care facilities; rest homes; or hospitals treating tuberculous patients. Exclusions may pertain to mental illness, attempted suicide, pregnancy and miscarriage, narcotics, and alcoholism.

Half of the state insurance regulators have taken action of some sort against mail-order health insurers. This action has ranged from sanctions against individual mail-order health insurance companies to broad advertising codes. The regulators have objected to advertising that emphasizes life-time or monthly maximum benefits when the daily benefit is more likely to be paid. Another complaint about advertising is failure to mention (1) statewide increases for policyholders that would increase individual rates, (2) restrictions for preexisting conditions, and (3) increases in rates after the first month. Also, the regulators have advised against advertisements intimating profit can be made by the ill subscriber. In addition, objections have been made to advertising limited enrollment periods when the insurers accept subscribers at all times.

The National Association of Insurance Commissioners has approved a broad, new advertising code for mail-order health insurance. All policy limitations must be stated negatively. Phrases such as "extra cash" would be prohibited. "No medical examination needed to enroll" may not be used when the policies have a limitation on preexisting conditions. Limited enrollment periods and reduced first month premiums would be eliminated.

There are three reasons why mail-order health insurance has many purchasers. First, mail-order insurers contend their benefits will pay the unreimbursed hospital charges of other health insurance plans. In most basic health insurance plans, there are costs to the subscriber that are not paid by the plans. These costs are advertised to be paid by mail-order insurance plans. Some of these costs are medications; nursing home care; private nursing services; and dental, X-ray, and laboratory services. These are the "other" costs that the subscriber must pay. Usually in health insurance plans, there are some gaps between hospital charges and medical fees and reimbursements.

The second reason for the popularity of mail-order health insurance is that the insurer advertises that household bills will be paid while the breadwinner is disabled. Mail-order health insurance does not pay for at-home recuperation. If a person is in the hospital 14 days and spends 3 months of recuperation at home, he receives only the benefits for 14 hospital days. Thus, there is no realistic disability protection.

The third reason why mail-order health insurance has many purchasers is that mail-order insurers advertise that the policies pay "other" health costs missed by other health insurance plans. Most mail-order insurers base their payments solely on the number of days a policyholder spends in the hospital. Eighty-four percent of the health care cost items are not linked to hospitalizations but to "other" charges and physicians fees.

Before the mail-order health insurance is purchased, the purchaser should realize the best buy is group health insurance. Nonprofit groups and commercial companies return more than 90 cents on the group dollar. Mail-order health insurance on individual policies, returned about 53 cents on the individual dollar.[7]

REFERENCES

1. Health Insurance Institute: 1972-73 Source Book of Health Insurance Data. New York, The Institute, 1973, 54 pp. Health Services and Mental Health Administration. United States Public Health Service: Current Estimates from the Health Interview Survey, United States, 1970. Data from the National Health Survey, Washington, D.C., U.S. Government Printing Office, 1972, 66 pp. Health Services and Mental Health Administration. United States Public Health Service: Acute Conditions. Incidence and Associated Disability. United States—July 1969-June 1970. Data from the National Health Survey. Washington, D.C., U.S. Government Printing Office, 1972, 65 pp.
2. Health Insurance Institute, op. cit., pp. 7-9.
3. Ibid., pp. 55-64.
4. Department of Health, Education, and Welfare. Social Security Administration: Your Medicare Handbook: Health Insurance Under Social Security. Washington, D.C., U.S. Government Printing Office, February, 1973, 31 pp.
5. Schoen, M. H.: Observation of Selected Dental Services Under Two Prepayment Mechanisms. Am. J. Public Health, 63:727, 1973.

6. Health Insurance Institute, *op. cit.*, pp. 14-16.
7. Mail-Order Health Insurance. Consumer Reports, *38*:304, 1973.

SUPPLEMENTAL READINGS

Arnold, M., Blankenship, V., and Hess, J. (Editors): Administering Health Systems. Issues and Perspectives. Chicago, Aldine-Atherton, 1971.
Ehrenreich, B., and Ehrenreich, J.: The American Health Empire: Power, Profits, and Politics. New York, Vintage Books, 1971.
Follmann, J. F., Jr.: Private Health Insurance. New York, Health Insurance Association of America, 1967.
Ginzberg, E., and Ostow, M.: Man, Money, and Medicine. New York, Columbia University Press, 1970.
Harmelin, W., and Osler, R. W.: Business Uses of Health Insurance. Revised Edition. Bryn Mawr, Pennsylvania, American College of Life Underwriters, 1969.
Hold, W., and Todd, Jerry D.: The Foundations of Life and Health Insurance. Austin, Texas, Bureau of Business Research, The University of Texas at Austin, 1971.
National Conference on Private Health Insurance. Conference Papers. Washington, D.C., U.S. Government Printing Office, 1968.
Reed, L. S., and Carr, W.: The Benefit Structure of Private Health Insurance. Washington, D.C., U.S. Government Printing Office, 1970.
Watson, G. N.: The Elements of Group Insurance. Revised Edition. Ontario, Canada, Institute of Chartered Life Underwriters of Canada, 1969.

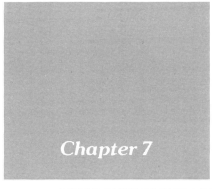

THE PHYSICIAN, DENTIST, NURSE, AND HOSPITAL

TODAY, there are numerous medical and dental specialities. There are quacks and charlatans "supposedly" treating the ill, injured, emotionally disturbed, aged, and poor, as revealed in Chapter 1. Too often, the patient may not know the differences in the professional preparation and functions of physicians, dentists, and nurses. This chapter will focus upon some of the professional preparation of, specializations within these three health services, and licensing of the physician, dentist, and nurse.

THE PHYSICIAN

Before the twentieth century most medical education in this country and in Europe was conducted through the preceptorial system. A physician interested in training a young man for the practice of medicine would accept a trainee. The physician would lend the trainee his books. He would teach the trainee about the anatomy and physiology of the human body, its diseases, and the treatment of those diseases. The trainee would serve as a general assistant. When the trainee completed his education, the physician would accept another young man under this preceptorial system.

Today most physicians receive their medical education in medical schools associated with large universities. States require that physicians licensed to practice medicine must be graduates of medical schools which meet the standards established by the Association of American Medical Colleges and the Council on Medical Education of the American Medical Association. Chiropractors are graduates of chiropractic colleges whose standards are not accepted by the Association of American Medical Colleges and by the Council on Medical Education of the American Medical Association.

There are more than 350,000 physicians in the United States or about one physician for every 640 potential patients. The desirable ratio is one physician for every 500 potential patients. In the Soviet Union there is one physician to every 420 patients. In Japan the ratio is one physician to every 900 patients, and in France the ratio is one physician to every 750 patients. In addition to the shortage of numbers of physicians in the United States, there is a decline in the number of general practitioners, internists, and pediatricians in relation to the U.S. population.

Americans who live in remote rural areas or in the inner cities have difficulty in obtaining adequate medical care. Rural counties with fewer than 10,000 residents may average one physician to every 2000 residents. Rural counties with 50,000 or more residents may have one physician for every 1000 potential patients. Many small communities, with the assistance of private foundations, have tried to replace physicians who have died or retired, but without much success. Many towns have offered to build small hospitals if physicians will establish their practices. Physicians seem to dislike rural areas because they are isolated from colleagues and sources of new professional information. Often they must turn their critically ill patients requiring hospitalization over to other physicians because of the lack of hospital facilities in rural areas.

In the inner cities, physicians move out because of crime, crowded clinics, ill-equipped hospitals, the "cultural gap," and advanced and more serious cases of illness than usual. Physicians making house calls take the risk of being robbed or seriously injured. Medical offices are tempting targets for thieves wanting narcotics. Crowded clinics and ill-equipped hospitals are found in the inner city. A "cultural gap" exists between some physicians and their black, oriental, Puerto Rican, Cuban, or Chicano patients, thus making it difficult to develop rapport between the physician and his patient. People living in the inner city may have more advanced and serious illnesses than residents in richer neighborhoods.

The number of hospital outpatients has doubled during the last ten years. Many outpatients could not get to see a physician anywhere else. Even in many prosperous suburban communities, physicians are so swamped with patients that they refuse to accept new patients. In addition, many patients with diseases such as tuberculosis are no longer hospitalized but are treated in outpatient clinics.

Four major objectives have been established by practitioners of modern medicine. First, good medical care must be available to all people. Second, the prevention of diseases must be given top priority and the patient must be kept healthy. Third, the whole patient must be treated, not just the parts of the patient as has been the tendency in some medical specialties. Fifth, reports of research into diseases and chronic health conditions and better methods of treatment must be continuously available.

Requirements for Admission to Schools of Medicine

The requirements for admission to schools of medicine are set by the Association of American Medical Colleges and the Council on Medical Education of the American Medical Association. Each school of medicine affiliated with a large university has a committee on admissions consisting of faculty who select the best qualified students. The prospective medical student should have at least 90 semester hours of academic courses such as one to two years of college English, two years of biological sciences, one year of physics, two years of chemistry equally divided between inorganic and organic chemistry, one-half year of mathematics including calculus, and other courses such as comparative vertebrate anatomy, embryology, genetics, bacteriology, and courses in the behavioral sciences. Applicants with less than a B average for all college work are not within the range for favorable consideration.

On most university campuses, there is a premedical advisory committee who can advise the prospective medical student of other required courses. Usually students are not accepted without three years of college work or 90 semester hours. Students between 20 and 30 years of age are preferred. Most students entering medical schools have earned a baccalaureate degree and have had four years of college work.

Approximately 11 to 16 months prior to the proposed date of matriculation, the prospective medical student may be required to take the Medical College Admission Test administered for the Association of American Medical Colleges by the Psychological Corporation, New York, N.Y. His score on this test becomes a part of his application and is one of the factors that will be considered by the committee on admissions. Applicants are selected by the committee on admissions on a competitive basis, and the best qualified are given first consideration. Personal qualifications, motivation for desiring to be a physician, scholarship, and probability of professional success are carefully judged. Personal interviews are required prior to acceptance and at the discretion of the committee on admissions.

A medical health data form must be filled out by the applicant to the medical school and by a licensed Doctor of Medicine. A dental health record must be completed by a Doctor of Dentistry.

Entering students are given a medical examination by members of the staff of the school of medicine. These examinations may be required at the beginning of each academic session or when requested.

Entering students may receive immunizations for the following diseases: smallpox, typhoid fever, tetanus, diphtheria, and poliomyelitis. However, they should have immunizations for smallpox, typhoid fever, and tetanus a year previous to entering medical school. The student must have a negative Schick test. A full course of diphtheria toxoid is given if the student is "Schick positive."

Most schools of medicine follow recommended acceptance procedures of the Association of American Medical Colleges. These procedures include time of matriculation, statement of intent, deposit of money which may be credited against tuition charges, application procedures, and appropriate regulations for accepted candidates.

The degree of Doctor of Medicine is awarded after satisfactory completion of the prescribed curriculum of the school of medicine. In addition, the candidate must be at least 21 years of age when the degree is awarded, have good moral character, have fulfilled all academic requirements, and have complied with all legal and financial requirements.

Curriculum

In most schools of medicine, the curriculum leading to the degree, Doctor of Medicine, takes four calendar years. Two curriculi will be described. These courses of study are similar to those in other first-rate medical schools.

The School of Medicine, Tulane University, a private, nonsectarian university, offers a 144-week program leading to the degree of Doctor of Medicine. This academic program takes four calendar years. In the first year, the student is required to take Anatomy, Biochemistry, Cell Structure and Function, Community Medicine, Correlation Conferences, Neural Sciences, Physiology, and two electives. In the second year, the student is required to enroll in Clinical Pathological Conference, Community Medicine including Biostatistics and Epidemiology, Correlation Conferences, Introduction to Clinical Medicine, Introduction to Clinical Topics, Laboratory to Clinical Medicine, Microbiology, Neurology, Parasitology, Pathology, Pediatrics, Pharmacology, Physical Diagnosis, Psychiatry, and two electives. During the third year, there are 12 weeks of Core Clerkships in Medicine, 12 weeks of Surgery, and 12 weeks of Pediatrics and Psychiatry-Neurology. The clerkship provides the student an opportunity to participate in direct responsibility for diagnosis and management of clinical problems of patients in the hospital. In the fourth year, there is a 12-week unit divided into eight weeks of Obstetrics-Gynecology and four weeks of Community Medicine, a six-week period of Outpatient Experience, a six-week period of Selected Advanced Studies in clinical or basic sciences, and 12 weeks of Selected Advanced Studies.[1]

The School of Medicine, The University of Texas Medical Branch at Galveston, a public, state-supported institution offers a curricular pattern of three major divisions: the Basic Science Core, Clinical Science Core, and Track Program. The Basic Science Core consists of basic science subjects formerly taught in the first two years of the medical curriculum plus Endocrinology, Cell Biology and Neuroscience, and two patient-related courses: Behavioral Science and Introduction to Clinical Medicine. The student has patient contact during his initial period of training. The Basic Science Core is scheduled in four 15-week periods, followed by a 10-week block of time for the course, Introduction to Clinical Medicine. In this course, the student rotates through various clinical services, develops his skill in performing medical examinations and learns the basic skills of diagnosis and the operation of the Medical Branch Hospitals. Some of the courses in the Basic Science Core are Gross Anatomy and Embryology, Microanatomy, Neuroscience, Biochemistry, Cell Biology, Physiology, Microbiology, Endocrinology, Pathology, Pharmacology, Integrated Functional Laboratory, Preventive Medicine and Community Health, Behavioral Science, Introduction to Clinical Medicine, and Radiology.

The Clinical Science Core consists of a 48-week period during which the student rotates through five major clinical services:

Internal medicine	12 weeks
Surgery	12 weeks
Obstetrics	8 weeks
Pediatrics	8 weeks
Psychiatry	8 weeks

The Clinical Science Core may include Neuropsychiatry, Obstetrics, Gynecology, Internal Medicine, Anesthesiology, Otolaryngology, Neurology, Ophthalmology, Dermatology, and Medical Jurisprudence. During the Clinical Science Core, a student must decide whether he desires to graduate following the Clinical Core. A student who elects to graduate, who is academically and personally qualified, and who obtains an approved university internship or residency is permitted to enter postgraduate preparation rather than to enroll in the Track Program.

The Track Program is a 48-week elective period in which the student selects from among three tracks: Medical-Surgical Specialities, Family Practice, and Academic Medicine-Medical Research. The minimum total time for the Track Program is 1920 clock hours.

The student who elects to graduate following the Clinical Science Core and who obtains an approved university internship or residency through the National Intern and Resident Matching Program will be permitted to enter postgraduate education rather than to enroll for the Track Program. The degree of Doctor of Medicine is awarded upon satisfactory completion of the first postgraduate year.[2]

Faculty

The faculty of Tulane School of Medicine includes more than 280 full-time physicians and professors. They are assisted in medical education by at least 720 part-time physicians and scientists. Tulane's medical faculty consistently has earned acclaim in research and education.[3]

The faculty of the 17 departments of The University of Texas Medical Branch at Galveston, School of Medicine consists of more than 539 physicians, professors, scientists, and full and part-time specialists in medical education. The School of Medicine is the eighth largest medical school in the United States and has a distinguished faculty which has received international recognition for research and education.[4]

Facilities

Most schools of medicine have access to several hospitals providing clinical service and teaching facilities and outpatient clinics. Other institutions such as research centers, institutes specializing in particular human diseases or defects, and psychiatric hospitals are close to schools of medicine. Hospitals must be approved for internships by the Council on Medical Education of the American Medical Association and for residents in the specialities of medicine. Hospitals must be approved for residency training in oral surgery by the Council on Dental Education of the American Dental Association.

Some of the physical facilities of schools of medicine include large auditoriums, lecture rooms, classrooms, class laboratories, research laboratories for faculty and graduate students, clinical and X-ray laboratories, faculty and administrative offices, poison control centers, dialysis center, clinical study areas, burns center, health defects center, family medicine areas, and rooms for publication of professional journals. There may be a special medical library building, a basic sciences building, clinical sciences building, graphic arts laboratory, medical television studio, computer center, museum of anatomy, and an overseas research unit. In addition, there are student health centers providing health services to students, counseling centers, physical education facilities, alumni headquarters, and book stores.

Libraries

Schools of medicine may have separate medical libraries or may share collections with local or state medical societies. Trained medical librarians are employed full-time in these libraries. Not only are there more than 2000 medical and scientific journals but also are there hundreds of thousands of books in the basic sciences, clinical medicine, allied health professions, and nonmedical fields. Often, these libraries have collections of the history of medicine, medical art, monographs, archival materials, and rare books. Special reading rooms, audiovisual centers, and research rooms may be found in these libraries.

Internship

After graduation from a school of medicine, the beginning physician may serve as an intern in a hospital for one year to prepare him for the state medical board examination. There are two types of internships. In the "Rotating" plan, the intern serves at least four months in internal medicine and eight months divided among surgery, pediatrics, and obstetrics-gynecology services. Or, the eight months may be in a specific service. In the "Straight" plan, the intern serves the entire year in a single service such as pediatrics.[5]

The intern's work is reviewed by a resident physician. The intern may examine a newly admitted patient, take a specimen of the patient's urine and a specimen of blood, make a tentative diagnosis, and may suggest therapy. His day may include "rounds" with an attending faculty member and a resident. He may do laboratory work and tentatively be in charge of the emergency room. He learns the skills of medicine from comments and actions of physicians with private practices, physicians who are faculty members of the medical school, and resident physicians. The intern attends formal lectures on the various medical specialities. If the intern examines a patient and makes an incorrect diagnosis, he is corrected by the physician and resident accompanying the intern. The correction is not done in the presence of the patient. If therapy by the intern is incorrect, the correction is made but not known to the patient. Upon completion of his internship, the intern takes the state board examination. If he passes the examination, the physician is licensed to practice medicine.

Residency

Most recent graduates of medical schools choose to go into a residency of two to five years in which the physician receives his specialty preparation. If the resident has chosen ophthalmology, the resident works in this medical speciality rather than circulating in the wards of the hospital as do the interns. As the resident works with patients who have been assigned to his specialty, he may supervise one or two interns undergoing preparation of the specialty. The resident is under the supervision of a staff physician who is usually on the faculty of a medical school. Often, staff physicians have private practices and teach in the schools of medicine.

State Board Examination

Before the Doctor of Medicine can practice medicine in the state where he resides, he must pass an examination prepared by the state board of medical examiners. The license to practice medicine is the official recognition that the physician has passed the examination. Reciprocal arrangements for the recognition of another state's license are found in a few states.

Medical Specialties

One of recent medical specialties approved by the Specialty Boards of Medicine is family practice. The American Board of Family Practice, Inc., was approved by the Liason Committee for the Specialty Boards. The American Board of Family Practice is a nonprofit organization, conducts examinations, and grants certificates to family physicians who meet qualifications and pass examinations. There are five purposes of the American Board of Family Practice. First, the Board seeks to improve the quality of medical care to the public. Second, it establishes and maintains high standards of excellence in the specialty of family practice and improves standards of medical education and facilities for this specialty. Third, the Board issues to licensed physicians certificates or other recognition of special knowledge in family practice and can suspend or revoke the certificates. Fourth, it determines by examination the fitness of specialists in family practice who shall apply for certificates and prepares and conducts such examinations. Fifth, the Board maintains a registry of those holding certificates and provides the public, physicians, hospitals, and medical schools with lists of diplomates who appear in the registry.

To be eligible for the specialty of family practice, the physician must have high moral and professional character. The physician must be a graduate of an approved medical school in the United States or Canada. If the physician is a graduate of a foreign medical school and licensed to practice medicine in United States prior to 1961, the physician must have a permanent certificate from the Educational Council of Foreign Medical Graduates. The physician must have a valid license to practice medicine in a state of the United States or a province of Canada in which the physician practices medicine. Last, the physician's eligibility is determined and established by the American Board of Family Practice and reviewed annually.[6]

The 28 medical specialties listed by the American Board of Medical Specialties are:

Allergy and Immunology—the medical specialty concerned with a hypersensitive state acquired through exposure to a particular allergen; study of immunity.

Anesthesiology—the study of anesthesia and anesthetics.

Colon and Rectal Surgery—the medical specialty dealing with diagnosis and treatment of diseases and disorders of the lower digestive tract.

Dermatology—the study of diseases of the skin and skin conditions resulting from diseases of the human body.

Family Practice—the Medical specialty concerned with the evaluation of a patient's or family's total health care needs, provision of personal medical care in one or more fields of medicine, and utilizing other health services needed by the patient.

Internal Medicine—the medical specialty dealing especially with the diagnosis and medical treatment of diseases and chronic health conditions of the internal structures of the human body.

Subspecialty—Allergy and Immunology.

Subspecialty—Cardiovascular Disease.

Subspecialty—Gastroenterology (study of the stomach and intestines and their diseases).

Subspecialty—Pulmonary Disease.

Neurological Surgery—the medical specialty concerned with surgery of the nervous system, both normal and in disease.

Nuclear Medicine—the medical specialty dealing with the application of radioactive material to the diagnosis and treatment of patients and study of human disease. The main tool of nuclear medicine is scintillography (introducing radioactive elements into the human body by injection or swallowing).

Obstetrics and Gynecology—the medical specialty dealing with prenatal care and all problems of pregnancy and childbirth; study of diseases of the female reproductive system.

Ophthalmology—the study of the diseases and disorders of the eye and vision.

Orthopaedic Surgery—the medical specialty concerned with treatment of diseases, fractures, and deformities of the bones and joints.

Otolaryngology—the study of the diseases of the ear and throat.

Pathology—the study of abnormalities of body fluids and tissues.

Pediatrics—the medical specialty concerned with diseases and chronic health conditions of children.

Subspecialty—Pediatric Allergy.

Subspecialty—Pediatric Cardiology.

Physical Medicine and Rehabilitation—the medical specialty employing physical agents (heat, cold, water, electricity, light, massage, manipulation, exercise, and mechanical means) in the diagnosis, treatment, and restoration of the convalescent.

Plastic Surgery—the medical specialty dealing with the reconstruction of tissues, particularly soft tissues, to relieve deformities, disfigurement, and malfunctions.

Preventive Medicine—the medical specialty emphasizing the control and prevention of diseases through research into their incidence and distribution and through public health measures.

Psychiatry and Neurology—the medical specialty concerned with the diagnosis and treatment of mental illness; the study of the nervous system, both normal and in disease.

Radiology—the medical specialty dealing with the application of radiation for both diagnosis and treatment of disease.

Surgery—the medical specialty concerned with the treatment of disease, wholly or in part, by manual operative procedures.

Thoracic Surgery—the medical specialty concerned with the treatment of diseases of the chest, wholly or in part, by manual operative procedures.

Urology—the study of diseases of the genitourinary system and male reproductive system.

The listings, but not descriptions, are from the American Board of Medical Specialties.[7]

Other specialties listed by other authors are Aviation Medicine (aerospace), Child Psychiatry, Diagnostic Radiology, Forensic Pathology, Occupational Medicine, Public Health, Therapeutic Radiology,[8] and Physiatrist.

Group Clinics

Group clinics or group practice consists of three or more full-time physicians formally organized to provide diagnosis, consultation, medical care, and treatment. In some group clinics, such as at Mayo Clinic, Rochester, Minnesota, or at Johns Hopkins in Baltimore, the number of physicians may be several hundred. Whether there are three or four physicians or several hundred physicians, the members of the group hope that by combining their skills and resources they can provide better services to their patients than they could individually. The group clinic provides opportunities for frequent consultations among the physicians and the pooling of laboratory and X-ray facilities. The large clinics offer residencies for young physicians preparing in the various specialities of medicine. Other advantages of the group clinics are (1) by sharing the patient load, the physicians may have more regular hours than the physician with a solo practice and (2) physicians are able to attend medical meetings, continuing education courses, and other activities. In 1973, there were more than 100 continuing education courses and at least 70 medical meetings scheduled in Texas.[9]

The group clinic may include family practitioners and specialists, or the group clinic may consist of different medical specialities or one medical speciality such as Internal Medicine. The physicians work cooperatively but remain individual physicians to their patients.

Charges for the physicians' services are established in a fixed schedule with some adjustment according to the patient's ability to pay. Most physicians have patients who pay little or nothing. Medicare, commercial health insurance companies, Workmen's compensation, Blue Cross, Blue Shield, or other health insurance plans pay at least some of the member's medical bills.

The monthly salary of the physician in the group clinic may be a percentage of the net earnings of the clinic or a contracted salary. The individual physician's salary is not directly related to the amount of money paid by his patient. In most instances monthly income of the clinic depends upon the payment of physicians' services by patients.

Choosing A Physician

When a person settles in a new community, he needs to select a family physician as soon as possible. Some persons choose their physicians from listings in the telephone directory, only to find that the physician is a medical specialist whom the person may not need. There are some questions which may be raised in choosing a family physician:

Is the physician (female or male) a graduate of an approved medical school?

Is the physician a member of the local, state, and national medical societies or associations?

Is the physician licensed to practice medicine in that state?

Is the physician involved in continuing education and medical conferences?

Is the physician a member of the staff of an approved hospital or does the physician practice at an approved hospital?

A telephone call to the local medical society or an approved hospital is usually an excellent means of obtaining answers to these questions. Or, a letter addressed to the hospital administrator might ask for a list of physicians on the hospital staff and their rank or level and surgical privileges. A physician may have staff privileges at several hospitals. When the physician is on the *consulting* staff of a hospital, he is an expert in his medical specialty and his advice is sought by other physicians. Physicians on the active staff of an approved hospital are physicians who spend most of their time at the hospital and are responsible for the medical care given in that hospital. Physicians who are *associate* staff of an approved hospital are physicians with less experience than active staff physicians. Often, these physicians are younger physicians. *Courtesy* staff physicians are physicians who can admit patients to an approved hospital but who do little work in the hospital. Courtesy staff physicians may not admit many patients in an approved hospital and may not be participating in the medical staff organization of the hospital.

Surgical privileges fall into three categories. A new physician interested in surgery may be granted *minor* privileges. The physician can perform operations and other medical treatments which have no chance of endangering the life of the patient. After performing numerous operations and being observed by other physicians, who are convinced that the physician has the necessary surgical skills, the physician is granted *intermediate* privileges. At this level of surgical privileges, the physician can perform operations that may cause some disability to a patient if the physician makes a mistake but would not endanger the patient's life. When the physician shows that he is competent at this level, he is granted *full* privileges. Now, he can perform operations that could result in serious disability or death to the patient if the surgery is done improperly. In an approved hospital, it may take a physician several years to reach full privileges. Also, if the physician is approved to do major abdominal surgery, he may not be approved for heart surgery.[10]

The local health department may have a list of community physicians, their ranks and surgical privileges. Public libraries have a *Directory of Medical Specialists*. If the new resident of the community is near a medical school, a telephone call to the medical school will provide the caller with the names of physicians with private practices who are medical specialists.

The physician's receptionist can give the hours of the physician's office appointments, his willingness to make night calls and home visits, and his willingness to accept consultation. Also, the receptionist can give the estimated fees for office appointments, night calls, home visits, laboratory tests, and hospital calls.

An office appointment with the physician will give evidence of his speech, manner, appearance, and his professional attitude toward his patient. The appearance and cleanliness of the physician's office and examining room will be seen. In the first office visit, the rapport between the physician and the patient is of great importance. The physician's sincere interest in his patient is often the means of building rapport.

Being an Intelligent Patient

Each patient should be aware that medical ethics binds the physician to respect the patient's confidences. Thus, the patient should fully inform the physician about signs that may indicate illness. Seeking the physician's services at early signs of illness will reduce hospital stays and physician's fees. The patient must be honest and truthful with the physician. When the physician has made the diagnosis and has prescribed therapy, the patient should follow recommended therapy. The patient should realize that a health record over a period of years gives the physician a broad base of information concerning the patient such as allergies to certain medications, results of laboratory tests, and results of annual medical examinations. If serious surgery is pending, the patient may wish an additional medical opinion. The patient should not hesitate to ask for consultation with another physician. Most physicians will welcome this consultation as an evaluation of their judgment. The patient should discuss fees frankly with the physician, particularly if payment is delayed or payment is in installments.

Above all, the patient should realize that the rapport between the patient and physician is based upon the desire to keep the patient healthy.

Foreign Physicians

A recent study sponsored by the Department of Health, Education, and Welfare has revealed that the United States is getting more new physicians from foreign medical schools than from American medical schools. One of every six physicians practicing in the United States as of 1971 received his preparation in medicine outside of the United States and Canada. One third of all staff doctors in American hospitals with graduate education programs in medicine are foreign-prepared physicians. These physicians total more than 63,000. Of this number, 25,000 received medical education in Europe, 21,000 came from the Phillipines, India, Korea, and other countries in Asia, 10,000 received medical education in Latin America, and 6,000 came from Canadian medical schools. Also, one half of the candidates for state licensing examinations are foreign-trained physicians. The study disclosed in the 1970–1971 school year that at least 13,500 applicants were refused admission to American medical schools. In 1971, although the medical schools of the United States had 8974 graduates, 10,540 foreign physicians were admitted to the United States, either as immigrants or as visitors, to receive specialist training.[11]

THE DENTIST

Today's practice of dentistry emphasizes the prevention of dental caries and periodontal diseases and early treatment of malocclusion. Even though the majority of dentists are general practitioners, the number of dental specialists is increasing. There are now eight specialties.

All types of "cures" for aching teeth have been promoted. One cure included biting off the head of a live mouse. Another cure recommended that the hollow of the tooth be filled with raven dung. It was even suggested that the teeth be touched by the hand of a corpse. A popular cure was to fill the mouth with cold water and sit on a hot stove. To rid themselves of the possibility of toothaches, some people purposely got rid of their healthy teeth. Soldiers in the mid-nineteenth century had to bite off the cartridges for their guns. If too many teeth were lost, the man was exempted from military duty. Other persons sold their teeth. It was not uncommon during the eighteenth century for a dentist to advertise his need to purchase healthy teeth.[12]

There are more than 8500 dentists in private practice in the United States and at least 1000 dentists in the armed services, United States Public Health Service, state health departments, large city public school systems, and the Veterans Administration. It is estimated that 20,000 dentists are needed in the 1970's in the United States. The Council on Dental Education of the American Dental Association accredits schools of dentistry for the preparation of dentists.

Dentistry has become a highly respected profession through efforts of dentists themselves. Standards of selection and preparation are continuously being evaluated. Sound professional ethics in dental practice have been emphasized.

Requirements for Admission to Schools of Dentistry

Students considering dentistry as a profession are advised to choose a program of study leading to the baccalaureate degree and to have an average of B or better in their overall course work. A grade of C or better must be earned in one year of college English, two years of biology of which one year is completed in residence and includes formal laboratory work, one year of physics, and two years of chemistry of which one year is general chemistry and one year is inorganic chemistry. All candidates are required to take the Dental Admission Test (DAT) by the Council on Dental Education of the American Dental Association. The DAT should be taken after the candidate has completed at least one year of predental college courses. DAT test scores are not accepted if the DAT was taken more than two years prior to the admission date.

Most universities have a preprofessional advisor who can suggest additional courses for the candidate to take in his predental college work. The candidate must comply with regulations as to his physical health such as having a medical examination given by a physician and a dental examination by a dentist. In most schools of dentistry, there is a committee on admissions which reviews the candidate's predental academic work, DAT scores, evaluations by preprofessional advisors or advisory committees, personal qualifications, motivation for desiring to be a dentist, and probability of professional success. Often, the candidate is required to have a personal interview with a member of the committee on admissions.

The degree of Doctor of Dental Surgery (DDS) or Doctor of Medical Dentistry (DMD) is awarded after completion of the prescribed curriculum of the school of dentistry and the candidate has been in residence so that this curriculum can be completed. In addition, the candidate must be at least 21 years of age and have good moral character. The candidate must complete satisfactorily a comprehensive examination in dentistry and must meet the academic standards required by the school of dentistry. He must have discharged all of his financial obligations to the school of dentistry.

Curriculum

In many schools of dentistry, an integrated multidisciplinary teaching program has replaced the traditional method of teaching departmental courses. In this program, clinical dentistry is available to the prospective dentist early in his preparation. The student has clinical experience in his first year and continues in the clinic throughout the four years. The basic science and supporting courses are continued throughout the four years. The achievement of each student is evaluated throughout his four years, including the clinical requirements of each department.

During the prospective dentist's first year, he may be enrolled in Cell and Tissue Biology, Human Biology, Developmental Biology, Applied Biology and Diagnosis, Prevention, Medical and Surgical Therapy, Restorative Therapy, Clinic Practice, and electives. In the second year, the student may have Human Biology, Developmental Biology, Applied Biology and Diagnosis, Prevention, Medical and Surgical Therapy, Restorative Therapy, Clinic Practice, and electives. In the third year, he may spend most of his study in different clinical practices: Preventive Medicine, Endodontics, Periodontics, Surgery, Unit Restorations, Fixed Multiple Restorations, and Removable Multiple Restorations. In addition, he may be enrolled in Developmental Biology, Applied Biology and Diagnosis, Prevention, Medical and Surgical Therapy, Restorative Therapy, and electives. In the fourth year, the student may have Applied Biology and Diagnosis; Prevention; Medical and Surgical Therapy; Restorative Therapy; Clinic Practice: Preventive Medicine, Endodontics, Periodontics, Surgery, Unit Restorations, Fixed Multiple Restorations, Removable Multiple Restorations, and Complete Restorations; and electives. At the end of the fourth year, the student may have completed 8 to 10 semester hours of electives. Courses in Cell and Tissue Biology include studies of morphology, biochemistry, biophysics, and physiology of cells and tissue during health and disease. Developmental Biology may refer to the growth and development of the human with emphasis on the behavioral and structural characteristics. Human Biology may investigate the studies of the organs and human physiology during health and disease. Applied Biology and Diagnosis may include studies of the accumulation, organization, evaluation, and application of knowledge to determine deviations from normal. Prevention may refer to studies which apply the principles of epidemiology, immunology, surgery, and therapy to control dysfunction or disease. Medical and Surgical Therapy may employ surgical principles and techniques on hard and soft tissue and administration of chemotherapy. Restorative Therapy includes those techniques employed to restore form and function to oral hard and soft tissues and construction and use of the prosthetic appliances.

Internship and Residencies

Following graduation, the dentist who wishes to complete an internship or residency usually has available various hospitals affiliated with the school of dentistry. These graduate programs are under the supervision of the faculty of the schools of dentistry.

Faculty

The faculty of schools of dentistry are dentists in general practice and dental specialists, scientists, physicians, pharmacists, and dental hygienists. These faculty members usually are hired on the basis of their research and education.

Facilities

The facilities for schools of dentistry usually include lecture rooms, seminar and conference rooms, classrooms, administrative and faculty offices, libraries, multiple and unit laboratories, television studios for closed circuit television, graduate and teaching research areas, and auditoriums. Each school of dentistry has clinical facilities. Clinical cubicles are provided for each junior and each senior student. Hospital facilities are available to schools of dentistry. In these hospital facilities, the dental student may observe surgical operations and hospital procedures. He may participate in dental surgery.

Libraries

Schools of dentistry have well-equipped libraries with full-time librarians. Volumes of medical and dental literature should be both up to date and broad in scope, serving the dental students, faculty, and dental practitioners in the community.

State Board Examination

Before the doctor of dental surgery can practice dentistry in the state where he resides, he must pass an examination prepared by the state board of dental examiners. Annual registration with the state board is required in some states. Reciprocal arrangements may be made so that a state board may accept the license issued in another state, but a practical examination may be required even though reciprocal arrangements are available.

Dental Specialties

The American Dental Association is responsible for the National Board of Dental Examiners. This Board gives written examinations similar to those of state boards. Some states accept these examinations in lieu of written state tests. All clinical and practical examinations are administered by state boards.

There is a nationally recognized examining board for each of the eight dental specialties. To become a diplomate of a specialty board, the candidate must have at least two years of advanced educational specialized preparation, meet certain other specific requirements, and pass a comprehensive examination.

The eight recognized dental specialties are defined as follows:

Dental Public Health deals with prevention and control of dental diseases and promotion of dental health in the community. The public health dentist is concerned with dental health education of the community, administration of group dental care programs, an applied dental research.

Endodontics is concerned with the prevention, diagnosis, and treatment of diseases and injuries that affect the interior tissues of the teeth, such as the pulp cavity. The endodontist treats infected root canals, removes diseased tissue through surgical procedures, and replants teeth that have been lost.

Oral Pathology deals with mouth diseases through the study of their causes and effects. The oral pathologist does not treat the disease itself but assists other dental and medical specialists by providing suggestions for effective therapy.

Oral Surgery is concerned with the diagnosis and surgery of the human jaw and adjoining structures needed as a result of diseases, injuries, and defects.

Orthodontics deals with the factors which control the growth processes of the teeth so that the teeth properly occlude. The orthodontist corrects malocclusion.

Pedodontics is the treatment of patients with different stages of dentition (deciduous, mixed, and young permanent). The pedodontist is concerned with the prevention and treatment of dental caries and periodontal diseases in children.

Periodontics deals with the diseases of the supporting structures (gums and bones) of the teeth. The periodontist treats patients with severe periodontal diseases.

Prosthodontics is concerned with the replacement of missing natural teeth. The prosthodontist makes artificial teeth or dentures.

Choosing a Dentist

When a person settles in a new community, he needs to select a family dentist as soon as possible. Several questions should be asked. Is the dentist a graduate of an approved dental school? Is the dentist licensed to practice dentistry in that state? Is the dentist a member of the local, state, and national dental societies or associations? Which dentists are general practitioners of dentistry or dental specialists? Often, a family physician, the local dental societies, and the local health department can supply the answers to these questions.

The dentist's receptionist can give the hours of dentist's office appointments. Also, the receptionist can give the estimate fees for certain dental services.

THE PROFESSIONAL NURSE

During the Crimean War, Florence Nightingale took a group of English nurses to Scutari to tend the wounded. She improved the care given soldiers in military hospitals. A few years later, the nursing services of Clara Barton during the Civil War brought recognition to American nurses and established nursing as a profession. In 1896, the American Nurses' Association was organized as the Nurses Associated Alumnae of the United States and Canada. The Association was incorporated in 1901 and the present name was adopted in 1911. Following ten years of study, the National League for Nursing was formed in 1952. The following organizations and committees voted to combine their programs and resources into the National League for Nursing: National League of Nursing Education, National Organization for Public Health Nursing, Association of Collegiate Schools of Nursing, and National Nursing Accrediting Services. The National League for Nursing is the accrediting agency for programs in nursing schools, which are usually located in the medical branches of large universities.

Programs in nursing schools include the Bachelor of Science in Nursing and the Master of Science in Nursing. The undergraduate program is planned for students who wish to enter the profession of nursing and who have earned a diploma in nursing and desire to continue in a degree program. The master's degree program is designed for those nurses who hold a baccalaureate degree in nursing and wish to prepare for positions in nursing service administration, supervision, or teaching in schools of nursing. However, there are nurses employed by boards of education, local and state health departments, college health centers, and industry who may have the Master of Science in Nursing.

Bachelor of Science in Nursing

Sixty semester hours of lower-division rank from any accredited junior or senior college or university must be completed from the following fields in order to enter the degree program:

Anatomy and Physiology	3 semester hours
Microbiology	3 semester hours

Electives in Natural Science	6 semester hours
Psychology	3 semester hours
Sociology	3 semester hours
Growth and Development	3 semester hours
History and Government	12 semester hours
Statistics	3 semester hours
English	6 semester hours
Free electives	18 semester hours

Two academic years precede the upper-division courses in nursing. Usually, a C or an overall grade point average of 2.0 must be earned in the lower-division required courses. A medical examination must be completed three months prior to enrollment in the upper-division nursing courses.

The University of Texas Nursing School (System-wide) is representative of programs for the degree of Bachelor of Science in Nursing. A total of 120 semester hours, of which 60 are in lower-division courses, must be completed. The 60 semester hours in the upper division are divided as follows:

Nursing Process: Care of the Well Individual	15 semester hours
Nursing of Individuals and Families with Minor Health Problems	12 semester hours
Nursing Intervention in Major Health Problems	12 semester hours
Nursing in Health Care Systems	12 semester hours
Electives	9 semester hours

In each clinical nursing course, the student must earn a minimum grade of C. A failed clinical course may be repeated only once and must be repeated in The University of Texas Nursing School (System-wide).

A student must have a C or 2.0 grade-point average on the 60 semester hours of upper-division nursing courses. The student must complete in residence 24 of the last 30 semester hours of the nursing major at the upper-division level in The University of Texas Nursing School (System-wide).

All senior students are required to take the Aptitude Test of the Undergraduate Program of the Educational Testing Service, Berkeley, California. The purposes of the test are to provide information on the student's competence and institutional self-evaluation.

Registered nurses who have no degree may transfer credit under policies of the Nursing School. Advanced standing examinations are given for previous preparation.

Master of Science in Nursing

The graduate curriculum includes courses for nurses who plan to teach nursing, who wish to be administrators, who are interested in medical-surgical nursing, who wish to be psychiatric nurses, and who plan to be maternity nurses. All students may have these courses: Fundamental of Research, Nursing Perspectives, and Thesis Seminar.

The University of Texas Nursing School requires two areas of specialization of all graduate students: (1) nursing administration or teaching and (2) clinical nursing. Clinical specialties offered are medical-surgical, psychiatric, and maternity and a combination of either medical-surgical or maternity with psychiatric nursing. Research Methods is required of all graduate students.

To earn the Master of Science degree in Nursing, the student must have 36 semester hours of upper-division and graduate courses, including a thesis, or 39 semester hours without a thesis. Only nine semester hours of upper-division rank may be included and may be taken outside the Nursing School depending upon the clinical and functional specialization. Students who elect the "thesis alternative" are required "to complete two courses, one in nursing and the other in nursing or a cognate area. In addition, one course must be either an advanced research course or an independent study course in nursing at the graduate level."

Before entering the program for the Master of Science degree in Nursing, the candidate must pass the Aptitude Test of the Graduate Record Examinations. The examination is taken at the candidate's own expense and during the dates established by the college or university administering the test.

An overall average of B and a B average in nursing courses are required. No grade lower than a B will be accepted in clinical nursing, teaching, or administration. A grade of C is permitted on courses meeting elective requirements.

All requirements for a master's degree should be completed within one six-year period. If the graduate work takes more than six years, those courses over the six-year period usually are not counted toward the degree.

Each graduate student must spend two semesters, or the equivalent, in residence at The University of Texas Graduate Nursing School. The student working on a thesis must be registered for the thesis course if that student wishes advice and assistance from a member of the faculty concerning the thesis.

Faculty

The faculty at The University of Texas Nursing School (System-wide) includes professional nurses with graduate degrees and specializations in nursing. In addition, some of these teachers hold administrative positions.

Facilities

Each nursing school has administrative offices, classrooms, lecture halls, libraries, study areas, educational media centers, and demonstration areas. Additional facilities for learning experiences include community hospitals which are general and private institutions, city-county hospitals, state hospitals, and armed forces hospitals. Community voluntary health agencies, local and county health departments, physicians' offices and clinics, state-wide referral centers for indigent patients, and community health centers are other facilities used in the undergraduate and graduate programs. At the University of Texas Nursing School components of the M.D. Anderson Hospital and Tumor Institute, Dental Schools, Graduate School of Biomedical Sciences, Medical Schools, School of Public Health, a mental health-mental retardation center, a county teaching hospital, a cerebral palsy treatment center, and a community guidance center are used.[13]

State Board Examination

Professional nurses may have earned the Bachelor of Science in Nursing or completed the diploma program. For licensure as a registered nurse, either by the degree or the diploma program, the nurse must pass the state board examination. All states and the District of Columbia require the nurse to have a license to practice professional nursing.

Specialties in Nursing

The registered professional nurse has many opportunities for employment in nursing.

Hospital Nursing.   Most hospital nurses begin as general duty nurses, working with all types of patients. With further education and experience, the nurse may choose to be a pediatric nurse, an obstetric nurse, a surgical nurse, a rehabilitation nurse, a nurse anesthetist, or a psychiatric nurse.

Nursing Education.   Nurse educators teach undergraduate and graduate students the principles and skills of nursing through classroom and bedside instruction.

Occupational Health Nursing.   The occupational health nurse provides emergency treatment for injuries and illnesses, assists in medical examinations, gives inoculations, keeps health records, and educates employees as to the prevention of diseases and accidents. The occupational health nurse works under the supervision of a physician.

Office Nursing.   The office nurse helps with the medical examinations of patients, gives immunizations and treatment prescribed by the physician, cares for and sterilizes instruments, and, at times, may do secretarial work in the physician's office.

Private-duty Nursing.   At the request of a family or a physician, the private-duty nurse provides bedside nursing care to home patients or hospitalized patients requiring continuous attention.

Public Health Nursing.   The public health nurse is employed by local, county, and state health departments and by the United States Public Health Service, and voluntary health agencies. The public health nurse is concerned with preventing illness, as well as caring for the ill. The nurse educates patients and their families about health problems and preventive measures.

School and College Nursing.   The school nurse is employed by the local board of education. The college nurse is employed by a college or university to work in its student health center. The school nurses may:

"1. participate in the in-service health services education of school personnel
 2. work with special education teachers on vision and hearing screening
 3. assist in the control of communicable diseases
 4. work with family and school physicians in developing efficient health services
 5. develop records for school nursing activities
 6. work with physicians, the superintendent of schools, and the health coordinator on exclusion and readmission procedures and on emergency care procedures
 7. work with school and family physicians on immunizations and tuberculin testing
 8. assist school counselors, the health coordinator, and teachers in discovering the emotionally disturbed child
 9. work with the Parent-Teacher Association on the readiness-for-school medical examinations
 10. assist teachers of health education and health coordinator in developing the total school health program."[14]

The most important functions of the school nurse are the home visits to educate parents as to the health needs of the student and the counseling of the secondary school student about his health problems. Several professional societies have published reports on the tasks of school nurses: School Nursing Committee of the American School Health Association; School Health Division of the American Alliance for Health, Physical Education, and Recreation; Department of School Nurses of the National Education Association; and the American Nurses' Association.

More than 700,000 registered nurses and 370,000 practical nurses are in the United States. Registered nurses were employed in the following facilities:

486,000   hospitals and nursing homes

51,000	public health departments and public schools
31,000	colleges and universities as nurse educators
20,000	industries as occupational health nurses
112,000	private duty, physician's offices, and other nursing specialties.[15]

Registered professional nurses are listed in nurses' registries: local, state, and national. Both registered and practical nurses are listed individually in the yellow pages of telephone directories.

Nurses and physicians are involved with a new approach to surgery—doing away with overnight stays in the hospital. Called "one-day surgery," "Verticare," "ambulatory surgery," and "same-day service," this surgery spares patients' nerves and pocketbooks. Some of the operations include removal of adenoids and tonsils, repair of simple hernias, biopsies, removal of noncancerous cysts and tumors, dilation and curettage, and replacement or repair of pins in damaged joints. Dentists provide oral surgery under general anesthesia.

The most common operations performed on a one-day basis are abortions. The majority of abortions are done in clinics or in hospital units that deal only with abortions.

Some of the criteria for permitting a patient to have one-day surgery are that the patient's general health must be relatively good, the area of the human body having surgery is limited in extent, the surgery can be completed in an hour, and the procedure is simple and can be done by a three-man medical team. In addition, there must be little chance of heavy bleeding or postoperative complications to the patient.

The patient who is scheduled for one-day surgery must follow a step-by-step routine. The day before the surgery, the usual laboratory tests are completed. The patient may not eat or drink anything after midnight preceding the surgery. Also, the patient is given medication to take the night before the surgery. At the hospital the next morning, the patient goes to a dressing room and changes into a hospital gown. An attendant takes the patient to the operating room. After surgery, the patient is taken to a recovery room and watched until he comes out of the anesthetic. When able, the patient dresses, goes to a special lounge, and is met by a friend or relative for the trip home. The physician may prescribe a sedative or tranquilizer to take on arrival at home. At a return visit for a checkup, the patient's bandages or stitches are removed. At least 1700 institutions in the United States now perform one-day procedures as a regular service.[16]

THE HOSPITAL

Hospitals may be classified as to the length of stay, type of patient treated, and ownership and control. The length of stay may be short term or long term. A short-term stay provides care for patients up to 30 days. At least 92 percent of all admissions are short term. The long-term stay is used by the patients with chronic health conditions, mental illness, severe disabilities from bone-shattering injuries, and some communicable diseases.

The type of patient treated may be general and special. A hospital treating *general* patients has these and other characteristics:

1. Maintains in-patient beds.
2. Has a governing authority legally responsible for conduct of the hospital.
3. Has an administrator who is responsible for the full-time operation of the institution.
4. Has an organized medical staff which delegates responsibility for maintaining proper standards of medical care.
5. Places each admitted patient for medical care under physician/ physicians of the medical staff.
6. Provides supervision by registered nurses and nursing services.
7. Maintains current and complete medical records for each patient.
8. Maintains a pharmacy whose services are supervised by a licensed pharmacist.
9. Provides diagnostic X-ray services with adequate facilities and professional staff.
10. Has clinical laboratory services with proper facilities and with medical technologists and pathologists.
11. Maintains complete operative room service with facilities and staff.
12. Prepares food to serve the nutritional needs of the patients and has special diets available.

The type of patients treated in *special* hospitals may have a medical, surgical, maternity, or convalescent problem or a chronic health condition. The medical problems involve physicians who are internists, psychiatrists, neurologists, and pediatricians. Or, the physicians may be treating patients with tuberculosis or venereal diseases. The hospitals having patients with chronic health conditions may be specifically for the care of the diabetic, epileptic, cerebral palsied, blind, or asthmatic.

The ownership and control of hospitals may be governmental or nongovernmental. The federal governmental hospitals may have patients from the armed services; Veterans Administration; the United States Public Health Service, such as, American Indians and Eskimos; patients with leprosy and narcotic addiction; and members of the U.S. Coast Guard and members of the U.S. Coast and Geodetic Surgery. Other governmental hospitals are state, county, and city hospitals. The nongovernmental hospitals are those operated by religious groups or fraternal orders and private (nonprofit) or proprietary (owned by individuals, groups, or corporations) hospitals.

Departments

There may be 11 departments within a hospital: the medical staff, nursing staff, dietary department, emergency service, laboratories, medical library, medical records, pharmacy, radiology, complementary departments, and nonmedical departments. The medical staff may consist of the chief of staff, chiefs of services, consulting medical staff, active medical staff, associate medical staff, courtesy medical staff, and resident medical staff.

The nursing staff has a director of nursing, supervisors, head nurses in charge of floors, general duty nurses, and practical nurses. Supervisors are responsible for the management of their sections, which includes requisition and maintenance of supplies, care of equipment, and nursing care of patients. Head nurses are responsible to the supervisors for the details of nursing care.

The dietary department must comply with standards from the Joint Commission on Accreditation of Hospitals. A qualified dietition must be employed on a full-time basis. Food service personnel and equipment for the storage, preparation, and serving of food are some of the features of this department. A systematic record of diets must be correlated with patients' medical records.

The emergency service should have a written plan for the care of mass casualties and be coordinated with the outpatient and inpatient services. Qualified personnel, adequate facilities, and complete medical records on each patient are essential to the proper functioning of this department. Accident victims, casualties of natural disasters, and indigents without family physicians may be treated in the emergency service.

Laboratories are divided into clinical pathology, blood bank, and pathologic anatomy. Clinical pathology examinations involve chemistry, bacteriology, hematology, serology, and clinical microscopy. Routine laboratory examinations on all admissions should be determined by the medical staff. The blood bank should have means of procuring blood, safekeeping of blood, and transfusion of blood. Pathologic anatomy involves examination of human tissues removed during operations. Reports of tissue examinations are filed with the patient's record, and duplicate copies are kept in the department.

The medical library must provide basic textbooks and current periodicals suitable to the needs of the medical, nursing, laboratory, and dietary staffs. A medical librarian and assistants should be available.

A medical record should be maintained on every patient admitted for care in the hospital. Medical records are kept confidential and retained for a period of time not less than that determined by the statute of limitations in the respective state. Qualified personnel should supervise activities in this department. Each patient is given a number upon admission. This number is carried upon all of the patient's documents which are filed according to this number. Clinical information shall be filed in the patient's record. Only members of the medical staff write patients' medical histories and medical examinations.

The pharmacy must be supervised by a registered pharmacist. Facilities shall be provided for the storage, safeguarding, preparation, and dispensing of drugs. Transactions of the pharmacy are recorded and correlated with hospital records. Special records must be kept as are required by law, e.g., prescriptions. Drugs dispensed must meet the standards of the *United States Pharmacopeia and Non-official Drugs*. Policies are established as to the administration of toxic or dangerous drugs with specific reference to the dosage and to the duration of use of the drug.

Radiologic services must be maintained according to the needs of the hospital. Radiologists and X-ray technicians promote services needed. Patients and personnel must not be exposed to radiation hazards. Radiologic examinations should be interpretated by physicians competent in radiology. Signed reports are filed with the patient's record and duplicate copies are kept in the department.

The needs of patients and the type of patient treated will determine if the following complementary departments are found in the hospital:

Department of Internal Medicine
Department of Psychiatry
Department of Surgery
Department of Obstetrics
Department of Anesthesia
Department of Dental Services
Department of Rehabilitation, Physical Therapy, and Occupational Therapy.

The nonmedical department consists of administration, admission office, special services, business manager, medical social service, and legal service. Among other functions, the admission office explains hospital rules to patients, discusses methods of payment with patients, sends patients to assigned hospital rooms, and notifies the physician of the patient's arrival. The special services may include the public relations director, volunteer program, and personnel director. The services handled by the business manager are information services, accounting office, laundry, housekeeping, and maintenance. Some of the activities of the medical social service are helping a patient who has difficulty in paying a bill, assisting a patient with a personal problem as a result of the patient's recovery, and helping the patient secure a job after discharge.

Accreditation

The Joint Commission on Accreditation of Hospitals is an independent voluntary nonprofit organization supported by the American College of Surgeons, American College of Physicians, American Hospital Association, and American Medical Association. Accreditation is voluntary and the hospital must be registered with the American Hospital Association, have at least 25 beds, and must be in operation at least 21 months. Requirements to be met for accreditation involve administration, construction and safety of physical plant, facilities, services, medical staff, nursing staff, dietary services, medical records, pharmacy, clinical departments, radiology department, emergency care for mass casualties, and medical library. There should be certain functioning committees for the accreditation such as credentials, joint conference (liaison between the administrator and medical staff), medical records, tissue, medical audit, utilization review (need for and length of hospitalization), infection review (possible sources of infection within hospital), and pharmaceutical and therapeutic.

Accreditation fulfills only minimal standards. An exceptionally outstanding hospital will provide patient care beyond the standards of accreditation. Accreditation is necessary for participation in Medicare.

Selection of a Hospital

With the assistance of the family physician or a medical specialist, the future patient needs to ask these questions:
Is the hospital accredited?
Is the hospital affiliated with a medical school?
Is the hospital large enough?
Who owns the hospital?
In addition, there are decisions to be made prior to hospital admission. Does the physician require the patient to be hospitalized? Can the ill person receive proper care in a nursing home or other health facility. What services such as a private-duty nurse are necessary for the ill person? How will the cost of the hospital services be financed?

In 1973, the American Hospital Association approved a "Patient's Bill of Rights." The patient has the right to:
1. Considerate and respectful care.
2. Complete and current information from his physician about diagnosis, treatment, and prognosis.
3. Information from his physician before treatment starts so that the patient can give an informed consent.
4. Refusal of treatment and acceptance of medical consequences of doing so.
5. Privacy in medical care including discreet conduct of examination and treatment and confidentiality in consultation, examination, and treatment.
6. Communications and records of his case which are confidential.
7. Reasonable response to request for services and transfer of case history to another institution, if necessary.

8. Information between his hospital and other health-care or educational institutions.
9. Knowledge of human experimentation affecting his case or treatment and right of refusal.
10. Reasonable continuity of care and health-care requirements after discharge.
11. Examination of his bill and explanation of it.
12. Knowledge of hospital rules and regulations while a patient.

These rights are expected to contribute to more effective patient care and greater patient satisfaction.[17]

REFERENCES

1. Tulune University Bulletin, 1972-1973, Tulane Medical Center: New Orleans, Tulane University, October, 1971, pp. 40-42.
2. The University of Texas Medical Branch at Galveston: School of Medicine Catalogue for 1971-1972 with Announcements for 1972-1973. Galveston, Texas, The University's Medical Branch at Galveston, 1971, pp. 91-94.
3. Tulane University Bulletin: op. cit., p. 8
4. The University of Texas Medical Branch at Galveston: op. cit., p. 14, pp. 102-138.
5. American Medical Association: Horizons Unlimited. Chicago, The Association, 1969, pp. 47-48.
6. Directory of Medical Specialists, Volume 1. 15th Edition. Chicago, Marquis Who's Who, 1972, pp. 155-156.
7. Ibid., p. v.
8. Hein, F. V., Farnsworth, D., and Richardson, C.: Living. 5th Edition. Chicago, Scott, Foresman and Company, 1970, p. 501.
9. 1973 Texas Continuing Education Directory for Physicians. Austin, Texas, The Regional Medical Program of Texas and The Texas Medical Association, 1973, p. 1.
10. McTaggart, A. C.: The Health Care Dilemma. Boston, Holbrook Press, Inc., 1971, pp. 36-37.
11. Flood of foreign doctors to U.S. U.S. News & World Report, 75:48, 1973.
12. Kogan, B. A.: Health—Man in a Changing Environment. New York, Harcourt, Brace & World, 1970, pp. 300-301.
13. The University of Texas Nursing School (System-wide). Austin: El Paso: Fort Worth: Galveston-Houston: San Antonio, 1972-1973. Austin, Texas, The University of Texas at Austin, 1973, pp. 7-49.
14. Haag, J. H.: School Health Program. 3rd Edition. Philadelphia, Lea & Febiger, 1972, p. 228.
15. Health Services & Mental Health Administration, U.S. Public Health Service. Health Resources Statistics. Washington, D.C., U.S. Government Printing Office, 1972, p. 170.
16. "One-Day Surgery" is spreading fast. U.S. News & World Report, 75:50, 1973.
17. Coniff, J. C. G.: How to tell a good hospital from a bad one. Today's Health, 51:42, 1973.

SUPPLEMENTAL READINGS

American Dental Association: Annual Report on Dental Education, 1972/73. Chicago, The Association, 1973.
American Medical Association: Survey of Medical Groups in the United States. Chicago, The Association, 1968.
Department of School Nurses, National Education Association: The School Nurse and Your Family. Washington, D.C.; The Association, 1971.

Freeman, R.: Community Health Nursing Practice. Philadelphia, W. B. Saunders Company, 1970.

Geyman, J.: The Modern Family Doctor and Changing Medical Practice. New York, Appleton-Century-Crofts, Inc., 1971.

Henderson, V.: The Nature of Nursing. New York, Macmillan Company, 1972.

National Council for School Nurses. School Nursing for the 70's: Washington, D.C., American Association for Health, Physical Education, and Recreation, 1972.

Rutstein, D.: The Coming Revolution in Medicine. Cambridge, Massachusetts, Massachusetts Institute of Technology, 1967.

Spalding, E. K., and Notter, L.: Professional Nursing. Philadelphia, J. B. Lippincott Company, 1970.

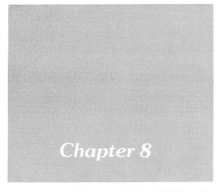

Chapter 8

PRESCRIPTION AND OVER-THE-COUNTER DRUGS

THE biggest channel of drug distribution in the United States is the legal, over-the counter (OTC) market available in drugstores, supermarkets, department stores, and news stands. The second channel is the prescription market which reached a total of more than 1.3 billion prescriptions at the beginning of the 1970's. Most of these prescriptions were antianxiety drugs. The black market was the third channel of drug distribution of amphetamines and other stimulants, barbiturates and other depressants, opiates, and small amounts of LSD and LSD-like drugs.

WHAT ABOUT DRUGS?

Drugs are substances used to diagnose, treat, and prevent illness. In the diagnosis of an illness, a patient can swallow a substance that will reveal on X-rays an abnormality in his intestines. Drugs can give relief from symptoms of a disease such as a fever. Antibiotics used in the treatment of diseases can kill specific types of bacteria. Vaccines such as the measles vaccine can prevent diseases.

Drugs can affect the functions of the human body. Morphine will depress the activities of the central nervous system. Aspirin may reduce moderate pain. Codeine can alter the sensation of pain. Oral contraceptive drugs can prevent ovulation and pregnancy. Drugs can control chronic health conditions, such as insulin controlling diabetes.

The amount of a drug taken can help or harm the person. Too much aspirin can kill a small child. An overdose of an anticoagulant may suppress blood clotting. Too many barbiturates with too much whiskey can kill a person. Antihistamines taken for hives may make the user sleepy.

Adverse or unfavorable reactions to drugs are drug side effects. All drugs have side effects. Some have mild effects while others have serious side effects. The physician should forewarn his patient as to the possibilities of these side effects and the importance of stopping the drug immediately if the signs appear. An adverse reaction may be due to the dosage of the drug, length of time the person has taken the drug, development of an allergy to the drug, or the user's general health. Some of the signs experienced by persons having side effects from a drug are weakness, dizziness, palpitations, shortness of breath, nervousness, loss of appetite, skin rash, pain in the chest or joints, sore throat, and bleeding. These reactions should be reported to the physician.

Safety and Effectiveness

The Food and Drug Administration (FDA) safeguards the public by requiring thorough testing of a drug for safety and effectiveness before the drug is allowed on the market. This safety and effectiveness are insured by the Federal Food, Drug, and Cosmetic Act, administered by the Food and Drug Administration. By law, pharmaceutical companies must present to the FDA adequate evidence as to the safety and effectiveness of new drugs before these drugs can be placed on sale. The pharmaceutical company must make extensive tests of the drug on animals and on human beings. The results of these tests are submitted to the FDA along with the names and qualifications of the investigators who tested the drug. A list of all ingredients and the amount of each ingredient in the formula of the drug must be given. There must be a description of manufacturing procedures and of all tests and checks made to assure purity and strength and to prevent errors in manufacture. In addition, qualifications of personnel who supervised the drug's manufacture must be stated. All labels and literature about the new drug must accompany the drug to be considered for approval by the FDA.

The results of animal and human testing and all other information about the drug are studied carefully by FDA pharmacologists, chemists, medical doctors, and other scientists. These experts must be convinced that the drug can be safely and effectively used and that the proposed labeling contains all necessary directions, warnings about possible side effects, precautions, and other information. If the FDA evaluation shows the drug to be safe and effective, it receives FDA clearance for marketing. Even after a drug is on the market, it may be recalled if there have been a significant number of people for whom the drug was not safe or effective.

If a drug is mislabeled, is contaminated, is improperly manufactured, or produces adverse reactions, the drug is recalled by the FDA and may become one of the Case Studies of Drug Recalls. The drug recall case studies indicate (1) clearly and concisely "what actually went wrong" in the manufacture of the drug and (2) what the pharmaceutical company did to correct and prevent errors of a similar nature from occurring in the future. Five steps take place in the case studies. First, there is the drug recall. Second, through cooperative inspection and investigation, the management of the pharmaceutical company and the FDA district personnel determine the basic reasons for the drug recall. Third, the FDA inspector prepares and submits a draft of a case study which describes the problem, its cause, and the measures taken by the pharmaceutical company to correct and prevent recurrence of the error. Fourth, the FDA selects and edits the case study to be published. Fifth, the case study is distributed as an educational and informational aid.[1]

Pharmacists may be asked if drugs deteriorate if stored a long time. Many drugs deteriorate and many become ineffective or dangerous when stored a long time. Over-the counter drugs should be dated when purchased. Prescription drugs will have a date given by the pharmacist. Some drugs have an expiration date and should be discarded when that date is reached. If a person is in doubt about the usability of a drug, he should dispose of it.

USP and NF

The first national pharmacopeia was published in 1820 as a result of the United States Pharmacopeial Convention called by a group of physicians who represented various state medical societies. The objectives of the convention were:

". . . to select from among substances which possess medicinal power. Those, the utility of which is most fully established and best understood, and to form from them preparations and compositions, in which their powers may be exerted to the greatest advantage. It should likewise distinguish those articles by convenient and definite names, such as may prevent trouble or uncertainty in the intercourse of physicians and apothecaries. The value of a Pharmacopeia depends upon the fidelity with which it conforms to the best state of medical knowledge of the day. Its usefulness depends upon the sanction it receives from the medical community and the public; and the extent to which it governs the language and practice of those for whose use it is intended."

The *United States Pharmacopeia* (USP) has four traditional functions: (1) selects the drug, (2) establishes names, (3) sets the standards and dosage forms, and (4) encourages physicians and pharmacists to use them. In 1820, the consortium which produced the first USP was entirely medical. Later, pharmacists joined in the work of revising the pharmacopeia. Today, the Convention includes representatives from every college of medicine and college of pharmacy, and state and national professional groups. In addition, seven agencies of the federal government are represented, including the Food and Drug Administration.

The *National Formulary* (NF), the second volume making up the "official" compendia, is published by the American Pharmaceutical Association. Its publication resulted from the need to standardize a large number of drugs that had not been selected for inclusion in the USP but nevertheless were being prescribed by physicians. The first NF issued in 1888 had extensively used dosage forms not described in the

USP as well as standardized names and formulas. At that time drugs were compounded largely by the individual pharmacist. Standardized formulations for preparing drug products were needed. In 1936, the NF reflected the modern trend toward large-scale pharmaceutical manufacturing. Before 1961 drugs were admitted to the NF according to their extent of use. The Board of the NF approved the present policy that drugs are admitted only on the basis of their recognized therapeutic values.

Both the USP and the NF use therapeutic merit as the basis for selecting drugs for inclusion in the compendia. Drugs selected for one compendium are not listed in the other. The USP is supported by the sale of its compendium and reference standards used by pharmaceutical manufacturers to check the quality of the manufacturer's products. The NF is supported by the American Pharmaceutical Association.

These compendia became legally "official" with the passage of the first federal Pure Food and Drug law in 1906. The FDA enforces the drug standards established by the compendia.[2]

Brand vs. Generic Drugs

The FDA's responsibilities for enforcement of the regulations for drugs are vested in the Bureau of Drugs which has more than 1000 personnel and a field force of 400 inspectors. Among the personnel in its highly technical bureau are at least 120 physicians, 100 microbiologists, 50 pharmacists and pharmacologists, and 50 chemists, plus statisticians, epidemiologists, and other professional personnel. The personnel of the Bureau of Drugs must complete a thorough assessment of a new drug or a drug recalled. Whenever a manufacturer wishes to market a chemical equivalent of a drug already approved by the FDA, the manufacturer must submit for FDA approval adequate data to demonstrate the equivalency of the product.

The Bureau of Drugs operates the National Center for Antibiotics Analysis and the National Center for Drug Analysis. These laboratories are designated for drug research and methodology development and for drug analysis. The National Center for Antibiotics Analysis is responsible for testing the potency, purity, and stability of *every* batch of *every* antibiotic before it is marketed in this country. If the samples meet all of the requirements, the batch is certified by the FDA. Only the certified batches can be released for marketing. Any manufacturer may decide to make the same certified product. This "me-too" product must meet all requirements of the original one. Each year the National Center for Antibiotics Analysis receives at least 20,000 samples for examination and 1.0 percent are rejected. The rejects cannot be marketed. From the years of experience with antibiotics analysis, "there is no significant difference between so-called generic and brand name antibiotic products on the American market. Any antibiotic offered for sale in the United

States, regardless of whether it is brand or generic, has met the same high FDA standards."[3]

Since 1970, the National Center for Drug Analysis has completed the study of 19 classes of drugs including adrenocorticosteroids, major and minor tranquilizers, urinary antibacterial agents, central nervous system depressants, antithyroid agents, cardiac glycosides, coronary vasodilators, anticoagulants, oral contraceptives, and others.

On the basis of data collected by the National Center for Drug Analysis, the Center "cannot conclude there is a significant difference in quality between the generic and brand name product tested." The National Center for Drug Analysis intends to publish data of the true picture on a given class of drugs. In 1972 the National Center recalled 638 drugs. Of these, 291 were brand name and 347 were generic products. Confusion as to the quality of drugs by the "big manufacturers," or "brand name," or "generic product" will be dispelled by publishing the results of FDA's national drug quality survey.[3]

IND and NDA

Investigational New Drugs (IND) and New Drug Applications (NDA) are handled by the FDA's Bureau of Drugs. Three testing phases of IND are required by the Bureau of Drugs to show that the pharmaceutical company has had "adequate and well-controlled investigations." In Phase I, pharmacology studies are used to determine toxicity, safe dosage range, preferred route of administration, metabolism absorption and elimination, and other pharmacological action. Small members of healthy volunteers are involved in these studies controlled by clinical pathologists. Phase II consists of initial trials on a limited number of patients with a specific disease or persons seeking prevention of a specific disease. Phase III requires extensive clinical trials to assess the drug's safety, desirable dosage, and effectiveness.

The IND form must include the following information:
1. Chemical and manufacturing data
2. Results of preclinical studies including animal investigations
3. Investigators' training and experience
4. Each investigator supplied with all informational material
5. Pharmaceutical company's agreement to notify the FDA about adverse drug effects
6. Consent of person to have drug tested on him
7. Agreement to submit annual reports and other data concerning drug when studies discontinued
8. Outline of planned investigation

The IND procedures must be clear-cut and meet other criteria. The outline or *protocol* can be the determining factor in approval of the IND application. After the three phases of IND testing have been completed, the manufacturer may file an NDA application.

The NDA approval will depend upon the IND protocol which must state a question or questions to be answered by the clinical trial. Second, the protocol must contain criteria for accurately defining and diagnosing the disease involved plus appropriate laboratory tests. The method of selecting patients and of allocating patients for treatment is the third factor of the protocol. The fourth factor is the elimination of bias by both observer and patient in reporting results of clinical trials. Fifth, the protocol should include steps to compare variables of sex, age, duration of disease, and use of other drugs not in the study. The methods used in analyzing the patient's responses are the sixth step. The nature of the control group against which the effects of the new treatment can be compared is the seventh step. Finally, the protocol must have a summary of statistical methods to be used in analyzing data from the patients.[4]

Falsification of Drug Data

The Scientific Investigations Group of the Food and Drug Administration has found that some physicians in charge of investigating new drugs turn in fictitious data to the sponsoring pharmaceutical companies. Inaccurate reporting of the studies, incomplete clinical trials, and using persons not aware of the testing are some of the items of the fabricated data. In one particular trial, two drugs were given to the same patients on the same days and in such a manner as to suggest that either one report on one drug or both reports on the two drugs were fabricated. In another drug test, mental patients were used without their understanding of the consent forms or knowledge of the drug experiment. Some consent forms were executed posthumously. Usually, failure to keep proper records and other administrative irregularities are found in falsification of drug data.

When falsification of drug data is discovered by the Scientific Investigations Group, criminal proceedings may be instituted against the physician investigator or his name may be removed from the list of official investigators. When the investigator is delisted, all pharmaceutical companies who have used the investigator must provide independent corroboration of the investigator's drug data. Recently the Scientific Investigations Group has been studying the records supporting the introduction of new drugs, rather than the investigator. Failure to keep or provide complete records of drug testing have resulted in 20 percent of the physicians being delisted as investigators.[5]

Manufacturing and Controls for IND's and NDA's

Existing regulations require new drugs to have proper identification, quality, purity, and strength. Additional information has been given to manufacturers so that they can complete the requirements in a satisfactory manner. In all IND submissions, there must be clinical pharma-

cology on a limited number of human patients. In addition, these guidelines are suggested:
1. Complete list of components in the drug including the new drug substance.
2. Quantitative composition of the drug, e.g., new dosage forms.
3. Source and preparation of the new drug substance, e.g., description of the synthesis.
4. Methods, controls, and facilities for manufacture of the new drug to establish and maintain standards of identity, strength, quality, and purity.
   a. Raw material controls include new drug substance and other ingredients.
   b. Manufacturing and processing, packaging, and labeling.
   c. Laboratory controls for final dosage forms.
   d. Stability of new drug substance.
   e. Batch control numbers explained.
5. Investigational label requirements.

The label for an IND should have "Caution: New Drug—Limited by Federal (or United States) law to investigational use."

The NDA submissions should list all components of the drug. Second, the quantitative composition of the new drug's dosage form should be stated in quantities of all active and inert ingredients per dose, e.g., per tablet. Third, all facilities and personnel of the pharmaceutical company must be completely described and can be determined by inspection of the pharmaceutical company. Fourth, a description of the method of preparation of the new drug substance must accompany all other requested information. This method of preparation provides another evaluation of the new drug. Fifth, proposed tests for raw material and specifications for the new drug substance must be submitted. Sixth, tests of the raw materials and specifications for inactive ingredients in the new drug substance should be included. Seventh, all procedures for manufacturing, processing, packaging, and labeling should be included. Eighth, the analytical controls, specifications, and test procedures for the finished drug must meet recommended standards. Ninth, a stability profile based upon studies must indicate whether the drug dosage form in its container will be suitably stable for the anticipated shelf life. Also, the suitability and safety of a plastic substance for use in a container must undergo test procedures. Tenth, instructions must be given as to the number of types of samples submitted.[6]

Microbiological Control of Drugs

During 1966, hospital outbreaks of bacterial infections occurred in Massachusetts, California, Oregon, and Ohio. In early 1967, an outbreak of a Klebsiella pneumoniae septicemia took place in a hospital in Worcester, Massachusetts. In 1967, the FDA found one manufacturer's nose drops and nasal sprays contaminated with bacteria. During a five-week period between July 30 and September 4, 1968, newborn infants in a hospital nursery had a hexachlorophene preparation used on them. Microorganisms of the family Pseudomonadaceae were found in all hexachlorophene containers.

The health hazards from microbial contamination of pharmaceutical and cosmetic preparations have created interest in the regulation of the cosmetic and pharmaceutical industries. The American Public Health Association, the Conference of State Sanitary Engineers, the Association of State and Territorial Health Officers, and colleges of pharmacy have joined with the FDA to suggest nationally uniform microbiological guidelines to reduce contamination in drugs.

Drugs for injection into the human body and solutions for intravenous administration must be sterile. Ophthalmic solutions and dispensers must be sterile to prevent eye infections. However, no such microbiological requirements have been in effect for baby powders, oils, and preparations used on the newborn. Also, such requirements have not been applied to hand and body lotions used in routine patient care in hospitals. Many varieties of bacteria, yeasts, and molds can cause fermentation, off-odors, decomposition, off-flavors, and discoloration of a product. Contamination of a product can be due to lack of sanitation during manufacture.

In recent years the pharmaceutical industry has developed procedures to prevent cross-contamination of drugs with antibiotics and other potent ingredients. Contamination of drugs can be due to raw materials, water supply, air supply, processing operations, equipment, employees, and environment and plant facilities.

Raw materials of animal or vegetable origin must be considered as a potentially higher risk than chemically pure products resulting from refining, synthesizing, or other processes where high heat, acidity, or alkalinity destroy microbiologic life. Water supply, both distilled and tap, should be checked frequently. Contamination from the microorganisms of the family Pseudomonadaceae has been found in distilled water supplies. The air supply of a pharmaceutical company can be contaminated with bacteria, particularly when large volumes of air are used for a spray-drying process. Air circulation patterns and systems, aerosols, and dust patterns must be considered for the possibility of contamination, cross-contamination and recontamination. Processing operations offer another possibility for microbiologic contamination. Another source of contamination may be the storing or holding conditions of the drug product. The cleaning, sanitation, and maintenance of equipment are another link in the control microbiologic organisms. A training program in basic sanitation and hygiene provided by the pharmaceutical company would help to control contamination among employees. The pharmaceutical plant may be located in a crowded industrial area where operations of other nearby industries generate dust, attract rats and birds, and have other undesirable environmental factors. The interior construction of the plant as to its floor drainage, cleanability, traffic patterns, and adequacy of sanitary features is important.

To control microbiological organisms in drugs, laboratory testing must be done on a continuous basis. This testing must take into account the nature of raw materials used, the physical nature of the drug, the moisture and nutrients available for microbial growth, the amount of handling of the drug, the use of the drug, and other factors that might enhance the growth of microbiological organisms.[7]

Drug Efficacy Study, 1962-1970

Thirty panels of physicians and dentists, experts in their specialties and selected by the National Academy of Sciences–National Research Council (NAS/NRC) Drug Efficacy Study Policy Advisory Committee forwarded to the FDA 2824 reports for 4349 drug products. Nine procedures were taken before the publication of the evaluation of the drug products. First, the medical staff, in consultation with pharmacologists and chemists, considered the Academy's evaluations in all reports pertaining to a given drug and to similar drugs. Second, a drug was classified as "effective," "probably effective," "possibly effective," "ineffective," or "ineffective as a fixed combination." Third, if the drug was effective, a decision had to be made whether an NDA or an abbreviated NDA will be required of manufacturers not now possessing an approved NDA. Fourth, methodology needed to be developed to assure equivalent patient benefit from different brands of a drug and from batches of the same brand of a drug. Fifth, as of February 1970, full labeling of a drug was not written by the medical staff when a drug was "effective" or "probably effective." Sixth, a list of all other approved NDA's or antibiotics was prepared. Seventh, after medical decisions were made, a proposed Federal Register notice was drafted to announce the effectiveness classification, the indications to be used in labeling, the period of time allowed for substantiating claims evaluated less than effective, and the conditions for marketing. Eighth, a letter and a copy of the NAS/NRC report were sent to each pharmaceutical company, whose drug was named in the study. Ninth, other manufacturers of the same or similar drugs were notified concerning their products.[8]

Ineffective Drugs

The Bureau of Drugs, FDA, continuously evaluates the findings of the NAS/NRC on the effectiveness or unfavorable benefits-to-risk rates of drugs. The 1962 Kefauver-Harris Amendments to the Food, Drug, and Cosmetic Act require that drugs be effective as well as safe.

The 1962 law applies to new drugs and drugs that came on the market through new drug procedures from 1938 to 1962.

In 1970 the FDA's Bureau of Drugs forwarded to all federal and state government drug procurement agencies a list of 359 drugs for which there was no substantial evidence of effectiveness or an unfavorable benefit-to-risk ratio. Some of these drugs have been removed from the market. Others are the subjects of actions contesting the FDA's findings. Some pharmaceutical houses are submitting data to establish the effectiveness of the drug product or making changes to render the drug acceptable.[9]

OVER-THE-COUNTER DRUGS

The Federal Food, Drug and Cosmetic Act divides drugs into two classes: over-the-counter drugs and prescription drugs. An over-the-counter drug (OTC) can be taken without a physician's supervision. The person using the over-the-counter drug, however, should read the labeling and reread the label directions each time the OTC drug is to be taken. The ingredients in OTC drugs usually cause few side effects when the drug is taken as instructed. The label must include:

1. Name of the product.
2. Name and address of the manufacturer, packer, or distributor.
3. Directions for safe use.
4. Cautions and warnings.
5. Established name of all ingredients.
6. Quantity of some of the active ingredients and of certain other ingredients.
7. Name, quantity, and specific warning for any habit-forming drug in the product.
8. Net contents.

A typical warning may tell the user how to use the OTC drug safely such as, "Do not drive," "Do not apply to broken skin." Or, the warning may tell the user when to stop taking the OTC drug such as, "Discontinue use if rapid pulse, dizziness, or blurring of vision occurs." The warning may read, "If pain persists for more than 10 days, consult a physician immediately." Any circular that comes with the OTC drug is also a part of the labeling.

There are at least 25 designated categories of OTC drugs:

1. Antacids
2. Antimicrobials
3. Sedatives and sleep aids
4. Analgesics
5. Cold remedies and antitussives (agents relieving coughs)
6. Antihistamines
7. Mouthwashes
8. Anti-infectives

9. Antirheumatics
10. Hematinics
11. Vitamins-minerals
12. Antiperspirants
13. Laxatives
14. Dentifrices and dental products
15. Sunburn treatments and preventives
16. Contraceptives
17. Stimulants
18. Hemorrhoidals
19. Antidiarrheals
20. Dandruff preparations
21. Bronchodilators and antiasthmatics
22. Antiemetics
23. Ophthalmics
24. Menstrual products
25. Emetics[10]

In advertising, the OTC drug is often called "proprietary" to distinguish it from the "ethical" (prescription) drug. The OTC or non-prescription drugs have the biggest market, since they are sold in drug stores, supermarkets, department stores, and news stands.

Proposed Standards for Safety, Effectiveness and Labeling of OTC Drugs

Estimates of the number of OTC drugs range from 100,000 to 500,000. These drugs present many problems to the FDA. For example, many OTC drugs are alike so that drugs from different manufacturers may contain identical or similar ingredients or combinations, although the dosage may be different. Many OTC drugs undergo frequent changes in formulations and labeling. Furthermore, a great number of OTC drugs have been exempt from the classification of new drugs.

To proceed legally against each of the thousands of OTC products on the market would require years. Sixteen years were necessary to take the word *liver* out of Carter's Little Liver Pills. Litigation against manufacturers of similar preparations would not be feasible, since some products would remain on the market and others would be introduced while competing products were removed. Inadequate consumer protection would occur where certain products would remain on the market.

The OTC Drug Products Evaluation had to be planned and conducted differently from that for prescription drugs due to many factors such as the problem of dealing with symptoms not necessarily traceable to any specific disease. Thus the FDA has had to deal with OTC drugs by establishing, defining, and describing therapeutic classes or categories of these drugs on an industry-wide basis and by means of a monograph. Those OTC drugs that meet standards of safety and effectiveness and are not misbranded, under recommended conditions of use for their category, may be marketed as before.

In the proposed standards for safety, effectiveness, and labeling of OTC drugs, there are certain guidelines:

1. Safety
   a. Low incidence of adverse reactions
   b. Adequate directions for use
   c. Warnings against unsafe use
   d. Proof of safety determined by adequate tests
   e. Published studies of the safety of the drug
2. Effectiveness
   a. Pharmacological effect of the drug to provide clinically significant relief to patient
   b. Proof of effectiveness determined by clinical investigations
   c. Investigations corroborated by controlled or uncontrolled studies, clinical studies, and reports of human experience
   d. Two or more safe and effective active ingredients combined in OTC drug
   e. Each active ingredient contributing to claimed effect
   f. Rational concurrent therapy provided for significant proportion of target population
3. Labeling
   a. Clear and truthful
   b. Not false or misleading
   c. Intended uses and results of the product
   d. Adequate directions for use
   e. Warnings against side effects and adverse reactions
   f. Easily read and understood
   g. Toxicity or other harmful effect prohibits sale[10]

Aspirin and Its Competitors

Retail sales of OTC drugs exceed $1 billion a year. Advertisers have been extremely successful in wooing consumers away from ordinary aspirin to buy new brands and subbrands of pain remedies. For every dollar spent on OTC drug pain relievers, more than 80 cents is spent on more costly competitors of ordinary aspirin.

Aspirin (acetylsalicylic acid) was first sold in Germany in 1899 and was accepted as a pain reliever. The German pharmaceutical company of Bayer patented aspirin in the United States. Until Bayer's patent expired in 1917, the American price of Bayer's aspirin was eleven times higher than the price in other countries.

After World War I, competing aspirin brands flooded the American market. To justify its higher price, an advertising campaign told buyers to insist on genuine Bayer aspirin. In 1934, the FTC challenged the

"Genuine Bayer Aspirin" campaign and the manufacturers of Bayer aspirin agreed to modify their advertising. The "quick relief" campaign was substituted. "For quick relief—always say 'Bayer' aspirin when you buy." To justify this statement, the consumer was urged to drop a Bayer tablet and another headache remedy into a glass of water. The Bayer tablet disintegrated faster than other headache remedies. Actually, this proved nothing. More than a decade ago, a noted drug expert disclosed that quickly disintegrating aspirin products were absorbed slower into the bloodstream. No recognized clinical studies reveal that a 5-grain tablet of Bayer aspirin relieves pain faster than any other 5-grain aspirin pain reliever.

The American Pharmaceutical Association reports that a combination of pain-relieving products has no clinical advantage over single component products. Thus, there is little increased therapeutic benefit to the patient. Bufferin has very small amounts of two common antacids that are claimed to prevent stomach upset. In 1971, the National Academy of Sciences—National Research Council challenged this claim. Its studies showed that Bufferin did not reduce the intensity or incidence of stomach upset any more than plain aspirin. Also, the studies disclosed that Bufferin was not absorbed any faster into the bloodstream than unbuffered aspirin nor "faster" nor "gentler" than straight aspirin.

Anacin contains numerous ingredients on the theory that if one ingredient doesn't work, several might. At first Anacin consisted of aspirin, acetenalid, and caffeine which the advertisements stated were "like a doctor's prescription." When acetenalid was proven to cause certain blood disturbances, Anacin substituted phenacetin. When phenacetin was linked to kidney problems, phenacetin was dropped. No evidence exists that caffeine is useful when combined with aspirin. Studies have shown that caffeine has no analgesic effect. Thus, the only significant ingredient in Anacin is aspirin. However, the Anacin advertisements claim that it is the "pain-reliever doctors recommend most for headaches." An Anacin tablet sells for three to six times more than ordinary aspirin and contains 6.17 grains of aspirin instead of the usual 5 grains.

Excedrin has four ingredients: aspirin, acetaminophen, salicylamide, and caffeine. Acetaminophen is an analgesic, relieves fever, and can be used by persons sensitive to aspirin. Salicylamide is less effective than aspirin for pain or fever when the same dose is taken. Also, studies have classified it as "not recommended" for use. One tablet of Excedrin has as much caffeine as a half cup of coffee. Yet Excedrin claims to be a "tension reliever" and an "antidepressant to help restore your spirits." It is estimated that Excedrin is no more effective than 5 grains of aspirin.

New OTC analgesics contain five ingredients instead of four. Vanquish has aspirin, acetaminophen, caffeine, and two antacids. Cope contains aspirin, caffeine, two antacids, and methapyrilene fumarate (antihistamine which has a mildly sedative effect). Arthritis Strength Bufferin contains 50 percent more of the same ingredients per tablet than Bufferin. In Excedrin P.M. methapyrilene fumarate (antihistamine) has replaced the caffeine in Excedrin.

The FDA has insisted that hazardous OTC drugs be adequately labeled. Ingredients such as acetenalid, the bromides, and aminopyrine have been eliminated from popular OTC products.

In August, 1972 the FTC had complaints against Bayer Aspirin, Bufferin, Anacin, Arthritis Pain Formula, Excedrin, Excedrin P.M., Cope, and Vanquish. The rulings on these complaints had two noteworthy aspects. In addition to refraining from false claims, the manufacturers must include in all advertisements relevant "affirmative disclosures." Corrective advertising must offset the false impressions from deceptive advertising in past years. Examples of corrective advertising would be:

"It has not been established that Bufferin is more effective than aspirin for the relief of minor pain."

"It has not been established that Bufferin will cause less gastric discomfort than will aspirin."

It was proposed that 25 percent of the advertising budgets for other products of these manufacturers would have to be devoted to corrective advertising for a period of two years.

Well-controlled studies have shown the effectiveness of aspirin. A Mayo clinic study compared plain aspirin with these products: acetaminophen, phenacetin, codeine, propoxyphene (Darvon), ethoheptazine (Zactane), and mefenamic acid (Ponstel). Neither patients nor physicians knew which drugs were used in the study. Some druglike capsules were placebos. Among the findings of the study:

1. No drug had significantly faster onset of relief or duration of relief than aspirin.
2. Side effects for aspirin were the same as for the placebo.
3. Aspirin led the list when it came to patients experiencing greater than 50 percent relief of pain.
4. Twenty-one percent of the patients using the placebo claimed more than 50 percent relief of pain.

For persons taking aspirin, the amount of aspirin should be monitored by a physician if the person has a chronic health condition. A full glass of water should be taken with aspirin. Some people are allergic to aspirin, and others experience mild stomach distress. Patients using anticoagulants should take aspirin under a physician's supervision. Persons with stomach ulcers should consult a physician before taking aspirin. No more than two or three tablets of aspirin should be taken at a time. The label's direction should be followed for children's doses.[11]

Vitamin E

The FDA has no evidence to support the extravagant claims for supplemental vitamin E. Some of these claims are that vitamin E will cure skin problems, ease arthritis pain, prevent ulcers, help grow hair, and increase sexual potency. Most people obtain the needed amount of vitamin E because many common foods contain this vitamin.

The Recommended Daily Dietary Allowance (RDDA) of vitamin E:

    4–5 International Units—infants
   10–12 International Units—adult women
     15 International Units—adult men and pregnant women

An International Unit is roughly equivalent to a milligram. The FDA uses the RDDA in its attempts to disprove the claims being made for vitamin E.

Even though numerous studies have shown the results of vitamin E deficiency in animals, these effects have not been found in adult humans. However, premature infants suffer from vitamin E deficiency which produces skin irritation and anemia. An extensive study of vitamin E was conducted for the Food and Nutrition Board, National Research Council, from 1953 to 1961. The investigation was to determine the effects of low levels of vitamin E on humans for six years. A group of patients at the Elgin State Hospital, Illinois, were subjected to tests to reveal any changes in their mental and physical health due to lowered levels of vitamin E in their diets. No apparent change was indicated.

Some medical experts claim that vitamin E helps patients with angina pectoris. Studies at Mount Sinai Hospital in New York, Duke University's School of Medicine in North Carolina, and the University of Manchester in England have shown that there is no evidence to support the efficacy of vitamin E in treating patients having angina pectoris.

Another contention is that low cholesterol or diets rich in polyunsaturated fats raise the body's need for vitamin E. Vegetable oil margarines contain 13 times more vitamin E than butter.

No evidence exists that normal or even excessive amounts of vitamin E are harmful. However, the FDA finds "no value in the consumption of any substance that offers no proven benefit."

Cosmetics containing vitamin E have been promoted for softening dry skin, erasing wrinkles, healing skin blemishes, and giving new life to aging skin. No evidence from controlled studies substantiates these claims. Also, the FDA has had no evidence that vitamin E is effective for use as or in a deodorant.[12]

Poison Prevention Packaging

Many OTC drugs and all prescription drugs are being marketed in packages that adults can open but most young children cannot. At least a half million children each year accidently poison themselves by eating fistfuls of aspirin or swallowing other substances and drugs found around the house.

The Poison Prevention Packaging Act became law on December 30, 1970. The law identifies the substances that should be sold in child-resistant packages and sets standards for the packaging. However, parents must buy products in new child-resistant packages, keep products in these packages, and close the packages after use.

All household packages of aspirin tablets had to have safety closures as of August 14, 1972, when shipped from the manufacturer. "The law does permit packaging of a single size in each product line in conventional containers for the benefit of the elderly and infirm."

By late 1972, oil of wintergreen and all drugs subject to the Narcotics and Dangerous Drug Act had to have the safety closures. During 1973, OTC drugs containing iron and all prescription drugs in oral dosage form were required to have safety closures. The physician or patient can request the prescriptions without safety closures.[13]

Hexachlorophene

Even though benefits as an antibacterial agent are available from hexachlorophene, there are risks. It has been used in creams, ointments, powders, toothpastes, cosmetics, antiperspirants, feminine deodorant sprays, mouthwashes, treatment of burns, and in showering and skin care.

Several studies have indicated the disadvantages of use of hexachlorophene. The first study revealed that hexachlorophene was found in the blood of burn patients when hexachlorophene was applied topically. The second study disclosed that hexachlorophene is absorbed through normal skin. Also, large doses of hexachlorophene affect the central nervous systems of humans and rats. The third study led to FDA regulatory restrictions of the use of hexachlorophene with human babies. Babies washed once daily with diluted hexachlorophene were reported as having absorbed hexachlorophene into their circulatory systems through normal, unbroken skin.

Following these studies, the FDA applied the "benefit-versus-risk" concept or placing all the evidence on a scale and weighing the benefits against the risks. Was the use of hexachlorophene in bathing hospital babies to prevent skin infections worth the risk of brain damage to these infants? The FDA recommended that total body bathing of infants with hexachlorophene be discontinued.

The American Academy of Pediatrics (AAP) announced a similar recommendation that the use of hexachlorophene for total body bathing of infants in hospital nurseries or at home be stopped. Also, the Academy indicated measures for controlling infections in hospital nurseries other than using hexachlorophene. Within a short time, reports concerning staphyloccocal infections in hospital nurseries which had discontinued hexachlorophene bathing flowed into the Center for Disease Control (CDC). Data from the hospitals concerning the infections were taken under consideration by the CDC, FDA, and AAP. These conclusions were drawn from the data:

1. Mild skin infections were reported in most of the hospital outbreaks.
2. No infectious outbreaks had been reported in hospitals having discontinued bathing infants with hexachlorophene.
3. Nurses and other hospital personnel had stopped washing their hands in 3.0 percent hexachlorophene before handling babies, contrary to FDA's recommendations.
4. Short-term, once daily bathing of infants in hexachlorophene should be considered if hospital infections were occurring. Babies were to be rinsed thoroughly after bathing with hexachlorophene.
5. If there was an outbreak of nursery staphylococcal infections, there should be reevaluation of hospital facilities and techniques.

Because hexachlorophene was widely used by the American consumer, the FDA proposed to limit the least important use of hexachlorophene in products purchased in supermarkets and pharmacies. Hexachlorophene-containing products were divided into three categories: drugs with small amounts of hexachlorophene, drugs with higher concentrations of hexachlorophene such as those to bathe babies in hospitals, and cosmetics. Drugs with small amounts of hexachlorophene, such as soaps, should be labeled: "Caution: Contains Hexachlorophene. For external washing only. Rinse thoroughly." Drugs with higher concentrations of hexachlorophene, such as a product containing more than ±0.75 percent, should be placed on a prescription basis. The FDA proposed that hexachlorophene be removed from cosmetics, except as a preservative in low levels. No more than 0.1 percent hexachlorophene could be used as a preservative and then only when other preservatives were not available.[14]

PRESCRIPTION DRUGS

A prescription drug is one that should be used only by the person for whom a physician prescribed the drug. The prescribed drug is designed for the patient and is based upon the patient's age, weight, general health, allergies, illness, and other factors. The Food, Drug, and Cosmetic law requires that the drug be sold only by prescription. A physician must write or telephone the prescription directly to the pharmacy, which must have the physician's written or telephoned prescription before filling the order. Prescriptions can be filled only by a registered pharmacist.

If the original prescription specifies refills, the patient can have the prescription refilled without checking with his physician. A pharmacist cannot refill the prescription without the physician's order.

The prescription drug label will contain the patient's name; name of the physician prescribing the drug; name, address, and telephone number of the pharmacy; prescription number given by the pharmacy; when and how often to take the drug; quantity to take each time; special instructions for use, e.g., "Take after meals"; and name of the drug. When writing the prescription, the physician tells the pharmacist what instructions are to be placed on the label. These instructions are to be followed exactly as given. If the label states, "Take three times a day," these instructions do not mean to take three tablets once a day. Usually the physician will tell the patient if the prescribed drug will cause the patient to become sleepy or lack muscular coordination.

The physician can write the prescription in three ways: (1) by generic name, (2) by trademark (brand name) chosen by the manufacturer to identify his product, and (3) by generic name with the manufacturer specified. If the physician prescribes by generic name only, he will write "tetracycline" on the prescription pad along with dosage instructions. If the physician prescribes the drug by its trademark, he has specified the drug and the manufacturer. Or, the physician can write the generic name, tetracycline, and the name of the pharmaceutical company whose product he prefers. Most of the time the physician will prescribe by writing the trademark because he may prefer a particular drug formulation, he has confidence in the competence of the pharmaceutical company, and he has had good experience with that prescribed drug. The physician knows the patient and his illness and the prescribed drug best for the patient. When the physician writes only the generic name, he authorizes the pharmacist to decide on the pharmaceutical company making the prescribed drug.

If the prescription calls for a specific brand of drug, the pharmacist must fill the prescription with that product. The pharmacist cannot substitute another product, even though the substitute contains the same basic drug ingredients. If the pharmacist does not have the drug prescribed by the physician, the pharmacist must obtain it or get the physician's permission to substitute. If the generic name of the drug and the pharmaceutical company are written on the prescription, the pharmacist must dispense that specific product. If the generic name alone is on the prescription, the pharmacist may select any formulation of that particular drug.

Drug Information Provided to Physicians

The Rx label or package insert is the document on or within most packages of prescription drugs. This insert includes indications, warnings, and other information relating to the drug's safety and efficacy. The insert is concerned with the uses for which a pharmaceutical company wishes to market a drug and is not intended to instruct the physician in his diagnosis or to replace the physician's education in pharmacology.

The prime example of Rx labeling is the package insert which includes all written, printed, or graphic material accompanying the drug while it is in interstate commerce. Catalogs, mailing pieces, brochures, and similar material distributed by pharmaceutical companies and containing drug information are considered as promotional labeling.

After World War II, dissemination of drug information to physicians became a major function of pharmaceutical companies. However, not until 1961 was the "Full Disclosure" regulation provided in the package insert. The package insert is a part of the pharmaceutical company's New Drug Application. Data from animal testing and premarketing clinical trials is submitted with the NDA.

The typical page insert is a single sheet of paper and has these headings: name, description, actions, indications, contraindications, warnings, precautions, adverse reactions, and dosage and administration. The name of the drug must include the established or generic name of the active components. Along with the chemical name may be the structural or graphic formula. Inert ingredients must be listed in all drugs other than oral drugs.

A physical-chemical description of the active components must be included. If the dosage has some bearing on the drug's effectiveness, this must be given. Data on melting point, solubility, and stability must be presented.

Actions reveal the pharmacologic effects in animals and man, including absorption, excretion, and metabolism. Indications for a drug's use are listed as specifically as possible. If the drug is for adjunct treatment, a statement to this effect may be required.

Absolute contraindications and strong relative contraindications are stated. Information is given if the drug is contraindicated in pregnancy. Warnings must be given if there are extraordinary hazards, dangers of treatment, special conditions, and important precautions. "Use in Pregnancy" is stated if the drug is safe for use during pregnancy.

Precautions indicate conditions to be observed in the use and administration of the drug under special and routine conditions. All known adverse reactions and those adverse reactions in which a causal relation is strongly probable must be given.

Included in the dosage and administration are the recommended dosage, frequency, routes, and duration of administration for various age groups and indications. Any difference in preparation and administration must be clearly stated if common labeling is used for one or more dosage forms or methods of administration.

Thus, when a physician receives a new prescription drug, the package insert contains data the pharmaceutical company has submitted to the Food and Drug Administration as proof that the drug is safe and effective.[15] Particularly is this true in the pregnancy statement and pediatric dose. When there is evidence of severe adverse effects in children from a prescription pediatric dose, there is a statement in the package insert that the drug is not recommended for children.

It is difficult for the FDA to establish without a doubt the safety of a drug for use during pregnancy, since the new drug is rarely tested on large numbers of pregnant women. Guidelines for animal reproduction studies have been established by the FDA to gather as much information as possible and to provide maximum safety data. The guidelines provide for a general study of "fertility and reproductive performance, teratologic and embryopathic potential, and prenatal and postnatal effects." The FDA recognizes that "animal experience cannot be used with certainty to predict human safety." The package insert will bear a statement of the safety of the drug in its use in pregnancy if the data from animal studies contain nothing significantly unfavorable. However, if results from use in animals are unfavorable and there is no human experience to contradict this or if there is insufficient information on human use, the drug is labeled contraindicated in pregnancy.

The FDA concern with the package insert does not end with its approval of a New Drug Application. The pharmaceutical company must submit a *supplemental* application to the original NDA when there is a major change in the production of the drug or a change in the manner of presenting the drug to the physician. Labeling changes are required by the FDA when there is adverse information about a new drug. Contraindications, warnings, precautions, or adverse reactions are placed on the package insert, or the drug is restricted as to its use.

Besides the package insert, there is the "Drug Information Bulletin" issued by the FDA and the "Dear Doctor" letter sent by pharmaceutical companies. Also, articles in medical journals and semimedical publications carry information about prescription drugs. Advertising and promotional labeling is the major source of information for many physicians. The *Physician's Desk Reference* (PDR), a type of promotional labeling, is used by physicians. Another source of information about adverse reactions or precautions is the pharmaceutical company's representative, or detail man.[16]

Prescription Drugs Not Available

The medical community has severely criticized the FDA for the lack of new prescription drugs to treat certain diseases and chronic

health conditions. Because of the delays of many years in the introduction of new drugs, there has been a sharp decline in the discovery
and testing of new and needed drugs. These new prescription drugs
are available in other countries and have been used in helping persons with asthma, high blood pressure, angina pectoris, arrhythmia,
tuberculosis, and mental illness.

By 1962, seven new prescription drugs for asthma had been introduced in Europe. By mid-1973, only two of these new drugs could
be prescribed by physicians in the United States. Persons with high
blood pressure and angina pectoris could not get a new prescription
drug available in Great Britain because it had not been approved
by the FDA. While ten prescription drugs to control arrhythmia
have been available in Europe, only one can be prescribed by physicians in the United States. Only 6 of the 47 new heart and circulatory medications introduced in other countries are available in this
country.

Studies have shown that 82 new prescription drugs adopted in
Great Britain and the United States between 1962 and 1971 were
available in the United States 2.8 years after they were available in
Great Britain. In 1968, a new antibiotic called Rifampin was used
to treat patients with tuberculosis in Italy. Scientific papers presented
before the American Lung Association showed the effectiveness of
Rifampin in patients whose tuberculosis was resistant to other antibiotics. Another drug was long-acting injectable form of tranquilizer
to treat schizophrenia developed by an American pharmaceutical
company and used in Great Britain in 1969. This tranquilizer was
not available in the United States until 1973.

Today, an NDA takes an average of 27.5 months to be approved
by the FDA. There are three main differences between the systems
of drug clearance in other countries and those in the United States.
First, the clinical testing of new drugs is longer in the United States.
Second, there are longer periods of investigations in the United
States. Third, thousands more patients are used in testing the new
drug in the United States. These time differences and the 27.5 months
clearance time account for the time lapse of new drugs introduced in
other countries and the United States. A drug undergoing testing
and clearance takes an average of seven years at a cost of $11 million
in the United States. From 1968 to 1973 no more than 13 new drugs
were marketed in the United States.[17]

Chloromycetin

According to the National Research Council, Chloromycetin should
not be prescribed for any disease except typhoid fever. Yet, this drug
has been and is being prescribed for millions of persons.

In the 1940's, Parke, Davis scientists discovered molds that yielded the antibiotic, chloramphenicol, which was effective in treating various diseases, including typhoid fever. The Parke, Davis research team learned how to produce chloramphenicol synthetically and bestowed the trade name, Chloromycetin on the drug. When introduced into the United States in 1949, it was accepted as a broad-spectrum antibiotic that had no adverse side effects. By 1951, Chloromycetin had helped to make Parke, Davis the world's largest pharmaceutical company.

In the June, 1952 issue of the *Journal of the American Medical Association*, an editorial revealed that aplastic anemia occurred in patients given chloromycetin. Even when it was administered in small doses, a severe blood abnormality appeared. Some deaths were reported. The editorial warned physicians to be on the alert for reactions among patients given Chloromycetin. At the same time, the FDA refused to approve any additional shipments of the drug, pending an investigation by a committee of the National Research Council. However, the FDA permitted the sale of Chloromycetin if it was carefully used by physicians in those fatal diseases in which its use was necessary. The FDA ordered a change in labeling to read, "Chloromycetin should not be used indiscriminately or for minor infections."

Sales of Chloromycetin dropped sharply. To counterattack this sales decline, a new sales strategy was tried. Detail men of Parke, Davis were to inform physicians that the FDA investigation gave unqualified sanction of Chloromycetin for all conditions for which the drug was previously used. Chloromycetin sales began to rise due to the marketing strategy, regardless of reports of adverse reactions in medical journals.

In the 1960 Kefauver hearings on the drug industry, it was revealed that the adverse reactions of Chloromycitin were minimized by detail men and that Parke, Davis had "watered down" warnings of the drug in direct-mail advertisements to physicians. Sales of Chloromycetin declined, and Parke, Davis was involved in 25 law suits about the drug. However, neither unfavorable publicity nor the threat of litigation about Chloromycetin could stop Parke, Davis from encouraging physicians to prescribe Chloromycetin. In 1962, Parke, Davis deleted from the *Physician's Desk Reference* all hazards of Chloromycetin and inserted a statement that the dosage, administration, contraindications, and precautions could be had from the package insert, detail men, or the company. The inserts were sent to the pharmacists and were not seen by the physicians.

The Kefauver-Harris act required all prescription drug advertisements to include a statement concerning possible side effects. The warning about side effects of Chloromycetin was obscured in a mass of fine print by Parke, Davis. In addition, the company ran a series of "reminder" advertisements, such as a picture of a bronchoscope in the Chloromycetin advertisements implying that the drug should be prescribed for respiratory infections.

In the 1968 Senate hearings, medical authorities testified that Chloromycetin had been prescribed unnecessarily in 90 percent of the cases. The *Journal of the American Medical Association* reported 288 cases of aplastic anemia of which 12 percent of the patients had been treated with Chloromycetin when they had common colds.

The evidence of the consequences of taking Chloromycetin is found throughout medical literature, yet some physicians prescribe the drug promiscuously. The FDA requires Chloromycetin advertisements and package inserts to carry a strong warning about its death-dealing side effects. The FDA requirement does not apply to Chloromycetin earmarked for foreign countries. Chloromycetin and similar chloramphenicol products parade under 43 trade names, many distributed abroad by Parke, Davis, its affiliates and subsidiaries.[18]

DRUG PRICING

Drug prices vary considerably in different locations of a city, town, county, state, and nation. Rent, insurance, shoplifting losses, employee salaries, maintenance and repair, and pharmaceutical supplies influence the cost of the prescription drug. In 1967 the American Medical Association revealed that the retail prices of identical drugs in the same city could vary as high as 1200 percent.

In 1970 Boston required all drugstores to post in the pharmacy the prices of most prescription drugs. Osco Drug, Inc., a retail chain in 17 states, became the first Boston drugstore to display prices of prescription drugs. It hired a market-research firm to measure consumer response to the price listing. Consumers were enthusiastic. In October, 1971, the Illinois Board of Pharmacy began to suspend the licenses of Osco pharmacists for displaying prices for prescription drugs. Other state boards of pharmacy in North Dakota, Iowa, South Dakota, Wisconsin, Idaho, and Montana took similar action or requested the price listing to be removed or the pharmacies closed for one day. Many pharmacists stopped giving customers' prescriptions to Osco pharmacists when the customers wished to transfer to Osco pharmacies. Pharmacy associations and state boards of pharmacy declared the Osco listing of prices for prescription drugs was illegal. Pharmacists resigned from Osco pharmacies and Osco pharmacies were not approved for apprentice training of pharmacy students.

The Code of Ethics of the American Pharmaceutical Association states:

"A pharmacist should not solicit professional practice by means of advertising or by methods inconsistent with his opportunity to advance his professional reputation through service to patients and to society."

The posting of prices of prescription drugs is considered inconsistent by the American Pharmaceutical Association only when the pharmacy lists other information, such as the total number of drugs available, delivery service, availability of emergency service when the pharmacy is closed, the pharmacy's professional fee, maintenance of a record of the patient's drug intake and side effects, availability of the pharmacist for consultation, and proportion of the prices of dosages to prices displayed in the pharmacy.

In 1968 the American Pharmaceutical Association stated that advertising prices of prescription drugs would cause consumers to compare prices in different pharmacies. This was considered wrong by the Association because it would cause (1) inefficiency in drug distribution, (2) physicians to prescribe needless drugs or larger quantities than necessary, (3) patients to use leftover drugs, (4) pharmacy profession to sink to the level of commercial sale of goods, and (5) no monitoring of patient's drug intake or adverse reaction to drugs. The Pennsylvania Supreme Court considered these arguments and struck down a Pennsylvania State Pharmacy Board regulation against listing of prescription drug prices. However, within a year, the Pennsylvania State Pharmacy Board put into effect a new regulation prohibiting pharmacies from advertising prescription prices without full disclosure of the prescription drug's contraindications, adverse reactions, actions, interactions, indications, and dosage.

Not only do state pharmacy laws and regulations inhibit advertising of prescription drug prices but they also control ownership, management, location, and hours of pharmacies. A drug chain may have to wait several years before obtaining a license from a state pharmacy board, the ownership of the drug chain may be questioned, the pharmacists of the drug chain may be harassed, the same pharmacists may be threatened with license suspensions, or pharmacy schools may blacklist the drug chain.

So that the customer can have a listing of the prices of prescription drugs, these suggestions are made. First, there should be repeal of state restrictions against advertising the prices of prescription drugs. Second, nonpharmacists or consumers should be appointed to state pharmacy boards. Third, there should be enforcement of laws, at the federal level and in most states, against false or misleading advertising of the prices of prescription drugs.[19]

REFERENCES

1. Early, R. D., and Nelson, G. W.: Case studies of drug recalls. FDA Papers, 3:22, 1969.
2. Bassen, J. L., and Beek, C. R.: FDA and the drug compendia. FDA Papers, 6:18, 1972.
3. Simmons, H. E.: Brand vs. generic drugs: it's only a matter of name. FDA Consumer, 7:5, 1973.
4. Finkel, M. J., and Zatman, J.: Investigational and new drugs. FDA Papers, 9:31, 1970.
5. Physicians who falsify drug data. Science, 180:1038, 1973.
6. Guidelines: Manufacturing and controls for IND's and NDA's. FDA Papers, 5:4, 1971.
7. Lennington, K. R.: Microbiological control of drugs. FDA Papers, 3:11, 1969.
8. Bryan, P. A., and Stern, L. H.: The drug efficacy study, 1962-1970. FDA Papers, 4:14, 1970.
9. Ineffective drugs. FDA Papers, 5:13, 1971.
10. Edwards, C. E.: Closing the gap: OTC drugs. FDA Papers, 6:4, 1972.
11. Aspirin and its competitors. Consumer Reports, 37:540, 1972.
12. Vitamin E—miracle or myth. FDA Consumer, 7:24, 1973.
13. Maisel, G. S.: Poison prevention packaging: new protection for children. FDA Consumer, 7:24, 1973.
14. Pines, W. L.: The hexachlorophene story. FDA Papers, 6:11, 1972.
15. Jennings, J.: The Rx label: basis for all prescribing information. FDA Papers, 1:10, 1967.
16. Ortiz, E. M.: Providing drug information to physicians. FDA Papers, 5:7, 1971.
17. Ross, W. S.: The medicines we need—but can't have. Reader's Digest, 52:97, 1973.
18. The peculiar success of Chloromycetin. Consumer Reports, 35:616, 1970.
19. Drug pricing and the Rx police state. Consumer Reports, 37:136, 1972.

SUPPLEMENTAL READINGS

Brecher, E. W.: Licit and Illicit Drugs. Mount Vernon, New York, Consumers Union, 1972.
Burack, R.: The New Handbook of Prescription Drugs. Revised Edition. New York, Pantheon Books, Inc., 1970.
Goodman, L. S., and Gilman, A.: The Pharmacological Basis of Therapeutics. 4th Edition. New York, Macmillan Company, 1970.
Houser, N.: Drugs: Facts on Their Use and Abuse. New York, Lothrop, Lee and Shepard Company, 1969.
Kreig, M.: Black Market Medicine. Englewood Cliffs, New Jersey, Prentice-Hall, Inc., 1967.
Lingeman, R. R.: Drugs from A to Z. New York, McGraw-Hill Book Company, 1974.
Mintz, M.: By Prescription Only. Revised Edition. Boston, Beacon Press, Inc., 1967.
Pearson, M.: The Million Dollar Bugs. New York, G. P. Putnam's Sons, 1969.
Takton, D.: The Great Vitamin Hoax. New York, Macmillan Company, 1968.
Task Force on Prescription Drugs, U.S. Department of Health, Education, and Welfare: The Drug Users. Washington, D.C., U.S. Government Printing Office, 1969.

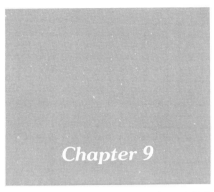

Chapter 9

CAREERS IN HEALTH PROFESSIONS

THE health professions suffer from a severe manpower and womanpower shortages in the United States and every country of the world. At the same time newly emerging health professions are developed by demands for health care and education of an individual, family, and community. Yet, the consumer is continuously confused by the many health professions, particularly when those professions are not the medical doctor, dentist, or professional nurse.

HEALTH SERVICE ORGANIZATIONS AND FACILITIES

At least nine types of organizations and facilities are the locations for the health professions. Local and state health departments, hospitals, mental health centers, industries and businesses, rehabilitation centers, research laboratories and institutes, elementary and secondary schools and institutions of higher learning, the United States Public Health Service and other governmental agencies, and voluntary health agencies and other related groups employ health or health-related personnel.

The local health department is the official health agency for a city or county. The city or county health department safeguards the purity of food and water; provides immunizations of all ages for various diseases; controls insects, rats, and other disease-carrying animals; prevents the spread of diseases by sewage treatment; monitors air pollution; educates the public on health maintenance and disease control; provides maternal and child health clinics; compiles health statistics; provides public health nursing services; offers some services for mental health and mental retardation; works with persons of different ethnic and economic groups in nutrition; provides laboratory other services dependent on the size and location of the city or county.

Each state has an official state health department. The state health department serves as a link between the local health department and the United States Public Health Service. The functions of the state health department differ greatly from functions of the local health department. Advisory and consultant services to the local health department are among the basic functions of the state health department.

The most familiar type of hospital is the community, general, and short-term which is supported by local taxes and hospital fees or is privately financed. These hospitals treat all ages and all kinds of illnesses and medical conditions. Some of the health personnel in hospitals are the administrative staff, physicians, nurses, orderlies, dietitians and food service workers, pharmacists, medical laboratory technicians, physical therapists, occupational therapists, clinical psychologists, housekeeping and maintenance staffs, recreational therapists, research scientists, and dental staff. The hospital provides services to patients, research, professional education, preventive services, and community health education.

Mental health centers are found in specialized hospitals, general hospitals, and community health facilities. The growth of mental health centers has increased with the public's realization that the mentally ill can receive treatment so that they can become useful members of the community. New kinds of drug therapy and other improvements in treatment have made the outlook for full or partial recovery from mental illness very encouraging.

Occupational health in industries and businesses is an accepted obligation of the management. The main concern of occupational health is to maintain the health of workers. An industry or business may have its own health services staff with a full- or part-time physician and a full-time registered nurse. In addition, there may be a safety engineer, sanitarian, and radiological health specialist. Accidents, overexposure to radiation, carbon monoxide poisoning, dermatitis, and the dust diseases such as silicosis are among the many occupational health hazards.

Rehabilitation centers may be found in the clinics of physicians, nurses, physical therapists, vocational rehabilitation counselors, orthotists and prosthetists, social workers, speech pathologists, audiologists, occupational therapists, and psychologists, to name a few. The purpose of rehabilitation centers is to help those disabled by accident or illness to become workers and useful family members. The disabled person may need therapy from many professionals to overcome or to compensate for the disability, education to prepare him for a suitable occupation, and guidance and assistance to get established in a job and keep it.

Research laboratories and institutes are not only in universities but also in hospitals and other places where health services are provided. Health-related research may be available in biomedical engineering, mathematics, psychology, sociology, economics, and business and public administration. Schools of medicine, dentistry, osteopathy, education, public health, nursing, and veterinary medicine are continuously doing research. State health departments and the United States Public Health Service have a range of research projects. Among the federal agencies contributing to health research are the Food and Drug Administration, United States Department of Agriculture, the National Aeronautics and Space Administration, the Environmental Health Administration, and consumer protection agencies (Chapter 10).

Elementary and secondary schools and institutions of higher learning provide jobs for school health educators, school nurses, school physicians, food service supervisors, corrective therapists, psychologists, college health educators, college physicians and nurses, and environmental health specialists. The school health program consists of school health services, healthful school living, and health education. In many states, health education is required in the total elementary and secondary school curriculum. The college health program may be focused on health services offered through student health centers and on environmental health. Health education in junior or community colleges, four-year colleges, and universities may be the basic college freshman health education course and the many undergraduate and graduate courses in school health education preparing teachers and administrators. In those universities with schools of public health, the faculty includes public health educators, administrators, statisticians, nutritionists, epidemiologists, and other personnel in public health. Education, research, communications, health maintenance, and public service are the main functions of the health professionals in the elementary and secondary schools and institutions of higher learning.

The United States Public Health Service and other governmental agencies focus on the health maintenance of all ages, research, education, and supportive services to the individual states. The United States Public Health Service is in the Department of Health, Education, and Welfare and has five agencies: Food and Drug Administration, National Institutes of Health, Health Resources Administration, Health Services Administration, and the Center for Disease Control.[1] Other governmental agencies are the United States Department of Agriculture, Office of Education and National Institute of Education,[2] Department of Housing and Urban Development, Department of the Interior, Department of Labor, Department of Justice, and the following independent agencies:
    Consumer Product Safety Commission

Environmental Protection Agency
Federal Trade Commission
Interstate Commerce Commission
National Science Foundation
Occupational Safety and Health Review Commission
United States Postal Service

In addition, there are other selected multilateral international organizations in which the United States participates, such as the Pan-American Health Organization.

The voluntary health agencies are financed by donations, gifts, and sales of published materials. Found in every state, these agencies include professional health workers and private citizens. Often these agencies identify health problems, educate the public to the problems, provide health services in those localities where the services are not available, and identify health womanpower and manpower needs. Some of the professional health workers are directors and field representatives, physicians, public and school health educators, health statisticians, social workers, and public health nurses. Among the voluntary health agencies are the American Lung Association, American Cancer Society, American National Red Cross, American Heart Association, National Mental Health Association, National Society for the Prevention of Blindness, National Foundation–March of Dimes, National Association of Hearing and Speech Agencies, National Easter Seal Society for Crippled Children and Adults, Planned Parenthood-World Population, and National Safety Association.

Other related groups are professional societies, youth groups, foundations, and commercial and semicommercial groups. In these related groups are found school and public health educators, health statisticians, information specialists, social workers, public relations directors, nutritionists, educators, physicians, nurses, and research workers. Among the professional groups are the American Medical Association, American Dental Association, American Nurses' Association, National League for Nursing, American School Health Association, American Public Health Association, American Dietetic Association, American Pharmaceutical Association, and American Alliance for Health, Physical Education, and Recreation. Among the youth groups are the 4-H Clubs, Future Farmers of America, Future Homemakers of America, Boy Scouts of America, Girl Scouts of America, American Junior Red Cross, Young Women's Christian Association, and Young Men's Christian Association. Usually, foundations are financed by legacies, trusts, or private grants of money. Foundations may provide research in many health-related fields. Commercial groups employ health professionals for many types of jobs in businesses and industries from the occupational nurse to the safety engineer, from the health educator to the health statistician, and from the dietitian to the food technologist. Semicommercial groups educate the public concerning health and consumer problems. Some of these groups are the Consumers Union, National Dairy Council, Cereal Institute, Good Housekeeping Institute, National Better Business Bureau, National Livestock and Meat Board, and Wheat Flour Institute.

EMERGING HEALTH PROFESSIONS

Each day new health occupations develop as the result of changes in job specifications or educational requirements, new training programs in schools, hospitals, and industries; and demands of the public. Some of these occupations are as an aide, a technician, or as an assistant, such as the physician's assistant. Many junior or community colleges, vocational and technical schools, hospitals, health departments, and private agencies, as well as four-year colleges, universities, and specialized schools such as schools of osteopathy, offer training in these emerging health professions:

Allergy environmentalist
Ambulance emergency technician
Cardiovascular technician
Child health associate
Computer operator
Dialysis assistant
Dietetic technician
Emergency health service worker
Environmental engineer
Extracorporeal circulation specialist
Genetic assistant
Geriatric assistant
Intravenous technician
Mental health worker
Nuclear medicine technician
Orthopedic assistant
Physician's assistant
Podiatric assistant
Radiopharmacist
Social rehabilitation service worker
Surgical aide

As computers continue compiling, analyzing, and summarizing health data, new jobs will emerge in the operation, maintenance, and repair of computers. In hospitals, automatic chemical analyzers, electronic devices, extracorporeal machines, and monitoring consoles will require persons skilled in their operation, maintenance, and repair.

The health professions are divided into seven groups:
1. Administrative, clerical, library, and health records personnel
2. Educators, information specialists, writers, and illustrators
3. Health specialists in the natural sciences, social scientists, social workers, and other health specialists
4. Other professional health workers
5. Sanitarians and engineers
6. Service specialists, workers, and aides
7. Technologists, technicians, hygienists, and assistants

ADMINISTRATIVE, CLERICAL, LIBRARY, AND HEALTH RECORDS PERSONNEL

Some of the health personnel in administrative positions are the local and state health officers, hospital administrator, executive director of a voluntary health agency, field representative, management specialist, public relations director, business manager, personnel director, purchasing agent, and admitting officer.

Local and State Health Officers

The administrators of the local and state health departments are physicians with specialized professional preparation and experience in public health. Some of the health officers' responsibilities are periodic appraisals of the community's or state's health needs, fact gathering and analysis of health data, provision of comprehensive health services, administration of direct services, and leadership for necessary teamwork among health workers in the local and state health departments. For each division or bureau of local and state health departments, there are directors, assistant directors, chiefs, and assistant chiefs.

Hospital Administrator

Responsible to the hospital's governing board, the hospital administrator is the person providing complete functioning and coordination of all of the hospital's services. The administrator must develop an effective team of the medical and nursing staffs, dietitians and food service workers, housekeeping and maintenance staffs, laboratory and pharmacy staffs, and other supporting workers. The administrator selects and supervises the staff members who are in charge of all departments. The hospital administrator must be able to cope with special emergencies, be aware of the community health needs and resources, carry out the broad policies governing hospital services, and administer the hospital with funds provided. In large hospitals, there are assistants and an administrator's executive staff. Usually, hospital administrators have completed graduate study in hospital administration.

Executive Director of a Voluntary Health Agency

A voluntary health agency usually focuses its attention on a particular health problem, such as cancer. The executive director administers the agency's activities, develops its program, organizes citizen committees for the agency's functions, works with local comprehensive health planning organizations, trains volunteer workers, takes responsibility for local fund raising, obtains information on local health problems, utilizes resources of the agency's national organization, and supervises the staff. In large voluntary health agencies, there are assistants to the executive director. Most executive directors of voluntary health agencies have completed graduate study in health education, public health, nursing, education, or business administration.

Field Representative

Most voluntary health agencies have field representatives who maintain contacts in local communities with the state or national headquarters of the voluntary health agency. Some field representatives work out of the national or state headquarter's office; others are found in regional offices. Some of the functions of field representatives are to serve as consultants to community agencies, provide communication between the national organization and local community agencies, bring national resources to assist with local problems, work with community leaders in establishment of a local agency, and administer a newly developed agency until an executive director is employed. Most field representatives have completed graduate studies in public health, community organization, or health education.

Management Specialist

With the expansion of health departments and voluntary agencies, the planning, coordination, direction, and evaluation of health programs may be done by management specialists. These personnel may be program analysts who are involved in the planning of the health program. Or, the specialist may be the program representative who goes into the community to interpret, implement, and expediate the program. Or, the specialist may compile facts, interpret research data, and promote citizen participation in new health services. Or, the specialist may be an administrative assistant on departmental administrative matters. Most management specialists have a bachelor's degree in public health, or health education, or public administration.

Public Relations Director

Public relations directors are employed by hospitals, voluntary health agencies, professional groups, commercial and semicommercial groups, and consumer protection agencies. The public relations director deals with many persons in a hospital—medical and nursing staffs, employees, volunteers, patients and their families, and visitors. Outside the hospital are the news media, community residents, and health departments and agencies. The public relations director must develop a communication program to help everyone understand the hospital's or the agency's services and goals. Some of the functions of the public relations director are to prepare informative booklets on services, produce a hospital or agency magazine, arrange tours and open house events, maintain good relations with news media, and offer suggestions for special programs explaining the hospital or agency services. Most public relations directors have a college degree with a major in public relations or journalism.

Business Manager

The business manager is the executive in charge of the business office of a hospital or health department. Some of the manager's functions include advising on financial policy, receiving and depositing all funds, payment of salaries and expenditures, and maintaining detailed records of all business transactions. The business manager has a bachelor's degree in accounting or business administration and post-college business experience in an accredited hospital. In a hospital, there may be a chief accountant, credit manager, and cashier who work with the business manager. The accountant reviews and prepares periodic financial reports including accounts of cash receipts, payroll and other expenditures, and patient accounts. The credit manager directs the hospital's credit and collection activities. The cashier receives payments from patients, maintains a working cash fund, prepares bank deposits, and may be a clerk, stenographer, or bookkeeper.

Personnel Director

The main function of a personnel director is to determine whether applicants have the qualifications and capacity for a particular job. The personnel director must analyze the duties of each position and have an understanding of how the job fits into the overall operation of a hospital, health department, industry or business, health agency, or educational institution. In addition, the personnel director is concerned with time schedules, pay scales, sick leave, vacations, and other fringe benefits. The personnel director should have a college degree with a major in personnel administration, business administration, or labor relations with at least one year of personnel experience. Assisting the personnel director may be an employment manager, employment interviewers, job analyst, training supervisor, and a salary and wage administrator.

Purchasing Agent

The purchasing agent buys equipment, supplies, and outside services; is familiar with the thousands of goods and services needed for operation; inspects products delivered; approves payment for those products; supervises storage; and issues supplies to the staff or workers. The purchasing agent must be able to evaluate goods and services. A high school diploma with emphasis on business arithmetic and bookkeeping is an important qualification. Assisting the purchasing agent may be a stockroom manager and stock clerks.

Admitting Officer

The hospital admitting officer and his assistants assign incoming patients to rooms and notify the proper hospital department of admissions. Up-to-the-minute records of room assignments, transfers, and departures must be kept. Most admitting officers have two years' experience in a hospital or social agency. Larger hospitals may have an assistant admitting officer and admitting clerks.

Director of Office Services

The office services include secretarial and typing services, bookkeeping and business machines operations, central files, telephone switchboard, duplicating, mail and messenger service, and receptionists. There may be a director of all office services or a chief typist, head bookkeeper, or an administrative secretary. Stenographers and clerks are assigned to various departments in a health agency, hospital, health department, business, or educational institution.

Director of Volunteer Services

In hospitals and voluntary health agencies, the director of volunteer services may provide in-service education for new volunteers, recruit volunteers, evaluate the volunteers' performances, and suggest ways to better utilize the volunteers' services. In a hospital, the volunteer may help with food trays and assist in some aspects of occupational therapy, music therapy, and recreational therapy. In a large volunteer program, there may be assistant directors. The director should have a college degree with a major in psychology, sociology, or management.

Medical Librarian

Medical libraries serve the needs of the professional staff (medical, scientific, administrative), professional schools (nursing, dentistry, public health, education), and hospital patients. Research scientists and all health professionals use medical libraries.

The medical librarian orders, classifies, indexes, and keeps files and loan records of the many materials in the library. In addition, the librarian searches for information on a particular subject, responds to mail or phone inquiries, assists in developing a professional school's curriculum, assists with hospital rehabilitation service, and provides recreational reading. The medical librarian must have a graduate degree in library science, good reading knowledge of foreign languages, and be certified by the Medical Library Association. There may be a chief librarian with assistants in charge of the separate library services, e.g., librarian in charge of the college of pharmacy's library.

Medical Records Administrator

Each patient in the hospital must have a complete, accurate, and continuous record from the time of admission to the time of discharge. This is the main responsibility of the medical records administrator. The data on the patient's medical record will include the patient's medical history, results of the medical examination, diagnosis, laboratory findings, medication, temperature readings, progress, and notes. Uniform medical terminology must be used in the medical records. The medical records administrator maintains all records in an efficient medical records library; follows a recognized classification system in coding diseases, operations, and other factors; indexes information from records; establishes catalogs; controls the use of records; and prepares medical and statistical reports. The medical records administrator should have a bachelor's degree in medical records administration or medical records science followed by the national registration examination. Assisting the medical records librarian is the medical records technician who does the technical work of maintaining medical records, reports, disease indexes, and statistics required in clinics and hospitals.

EDUCATORS, INFORMATION SPECIALISTS, WRITERS, AND ILLUSTRATORS

In this group are the school and public health educators, health information specialists, computer programers and operators, science and technical writers, and medical illustrators.

School Health Educator

Found in secondary schools, junior or community colleges, and those colleges and universities with teacher education programs, the school health educator teaches health education in regularly scheduled courses and assists in the development of school and college health programs. In secondary schools, the subject matter includes the 13 areas of health education: care of all parts of the human body; prevention of diseases; chronic health conditions; American Red Cross First Aid;

safety education; mental health; nutrition; community health; consumer health; adult health problems; family life and sex education; drug abuse, narcotic addiction, smoking, and misuse of alcoholic beverages; and international health.[4] In junior and senior colleges, the subject matter involves the basic freshman health education course; the professional courses in health education which focus upon teacher education; community health education; and health education courses designed to supplement the preparation of nurses, physicians, dentists, pharmacists, and other health professionals. These health educators should have bachelor's and master's degrees with major emphasis in school health education and teacher certification as required by most states.

In many school systems, health education is taught from kindergarten through grade 12. A supervisor or consultant of health education assists elementary school classroom teachers and those teachers assigned health education in the secondary schools to provide health education which fits the students' health needs. The school health coordinator works with the superintendent of schools, school nurses and physicians, and other school and community personnel in organizing and administering the total school health program. These supervisors and coordinators must have completed graduate study in school health education and in educational administration or supervision, have public school experiences as teachers of health education, and have teacher certification as supervisors or administrators.

Professors of school health education are found in colleges and universities granting baccalaureate and graduate degrees. These professors prepare teachers of health education for the secondary schools, consultants or supervisors of health education, health coordinators, future professors of school health education, and the following school personnel in their tasks in the total school health program: elementary school classroom teachers, school nurses, physical educators, special education teachers, and school administrators. Professors of school health education have earned doctorates with specialization in school health education, should have public school experiences as teachers or supervisors of health education, and have certification in school health education from a state teacher certification agency.[5]

Public Health Educator

The main function of the public health educator is to educate those persons not attending public schools and colleges about health so that they can protect their well-being and that of their families. Public health educators are employed by local and state health departments, the United States Public Health Service, voluntary health agencies, and universities preparing public health educators. These health educators work with other members of local and state health departments, community group leaders, executives and union members of industries, leaders of ethnic groups, and the news media. The public health educator stimulates people in the community to recognize their health problems and to solve these problems. He must be able to use many different methods of communication and be an expert in working with an individual, group, and community. Often, he provides in-service training for food handlers, sanitarians, volunteers in community projects, and certain health professionals not acquainted with ethnic or cultural patterns. In those universities with schools of public health, there may be programs with specialization in public health education and with graduate degrees in public health.

Health Information Specialist

Employed by voluntary health agencies and state health departments, the health information specialist is the news link between the health organization and the public. Life insurance companies and foundations employ these specialists, too. In a large organization, the health information specialist heads a department or section of public information with certain staff members with responsibility for one particular channel of information, e.g., television. Other staff members may prepare pamphlets, abstract information, and produce film-strips. The specialist must have the ability to communicate effectively, have up-to-date health information, and reach all segments of the community. The health information specialist should have a bachelor's degree in journalism with supplementary study in health education.

Computer Programers and Operators

In many hospitals, health agencies and departments, educational institutions, businesses and industries, research institutes, and government agencies, computer programers and operators take health data and supply the particular information wanted. Medical examinations, accident statistics, medical or health records, birth and death statistics, financial accounts, cancer fatalities, students' records, library information, research data, personnel records, insurance statistics, and morbidity statistics are some of the data fed into computers. As more health data are compiled, computer programers and operators will be needed.

Science and Technical Writers

Science writers are experienced journalists who specialize in medicine and health-related fields. They may write for magazines, newspapers, professional publications, radio, and television. They not only report what is occurring in the health professions but also interpret the information, e.g., a new treatment for heart disease. They explain new and complex health information in readily understandable terms. Science writers interview many health professionals and must be able to present the facts objectively and accurately. A bachelor's degree with major concentration in journalism and supplementary courses in health education are advisable academic qualifications.

Technical writers focus their writing about scientific developments for the professionals in the health fields. Technical writers prepare publications, reports, descriptions of new or proposed research, instructions for new instrumentation, and reports of proceedings of scientific meetings. They may prepare manuals for laboratory technicians, contract proposals for research workers, and specifications used in the manufacture of a new drug. Since technical writers must present accurate and detailed information for readers who are familiar with a subject, these writers must have a substantial background of technical information on the subject about which they intend to write. Technical writers need a bachelor of science degree in one of the basic sciences with a minor in journalism or a bachelor of arts degree in English with a minor in the basic sciences. Supplementary study in health education would be desirable. Technical writers are employed by scientific and medical publishers, manufacturers, professional societies, health agencies, universities, foundations, and governmental agencies.

Medical Illustrator

The types of visual presentations used by the medical illustrator are drawings, charts and graphs, models, animated slides and film strips, photography, exhibits, and television. Many illustrators become specialists, such as those who prepare drawings of the structures of the human body for publications in medical education. The illustrator provides the health professions with visual presentations of various types of surgery, cell structure, functioning of the heart muscles, procedures used by physical therapists, progress of dental decay, nursing techniques, and procedures of food technologists. The art media may be water color, crayon, pen and ink, air brush, pencil, wax, plaster, or plastics. The medical illustrator should have extensive college preparation in art and the biological sciences.

HEALTH SPECIALISTS IN THE NATURAL SCIENCES, SOCIAL SCIENTISTS, SOCIAL WORKERS, AND OTHER HEALTH SPECIALISTS

In this division of the health professions will be found the health specialists in the natural sciences such as the biochemist, bacteriologist and microbiologist, geneticist, pharmacologist, virologist, hematologist, and biophysicist. In addition, there will be the biomathematician and the social scientists—psychologist, psychometrist, sociologist, health economist, medical social worker, and psychiatric social worker. Other health specialists are the public health statistician, rehabilitation counselor, radiologic health specialist, and food and drug inspector and analyst.

Biochemist and Other Scientists

The biochemist reveals the chemical processes necessary for the cell's nutrition, growth, and reproduction and influence of various illnesses on these processes. For example, the nutritional deficiencies of the human body are influenced by human biochemistry. The bacteriologist and microbiologist disclose how microscopic organisms invade human cells and cause disease. The geneticist probes into the hereditary aspects of diabetes, epilepsy, sickle cell anemia, rheumatic fever, muscular dystrophy, cancer and other disorders. The pharmacologist discloses the healing and curative effects of drugs and medications and the poisonous effects of some drugs on tissues and organs of the human body. The virologist studies how viruses originate, grow and multiply, and affect living tissues, as well as how to prepare vaccines to protect the human body against these viruses. The hematologist specializes in the diseases and defects of the blood and blood-forming organs, such as anemia. The biophysicist is concerned with how the human body creates and uses energy, how nerve impulses are transmitted through the nervous system, how the eyes and ears receive and transmit light and sound waves, how muscle fibers respond to various stimuli, and which neurologic processes take place in thinking, feeling, and memory. Specialized areas of biophysics are radiologic physics (effects of radiation on living structures and tissues and the potential hazards of the radiation), cryogenics (low-temperature physics), and hydrostatics (physics of liquids).

Biomathematician

The biomathematician applies mathematical principles to the life sciences. By the use of mathematical models, the biomathematician explains life processes that cannot be demonstrated efficiently in the laboratory. He works with the epidemiologist who investigates various factors and conditions that determine the occurrence and distribution of disease, defect, disability, health, and death among the population.

Social Scientists

Among the social scientists are the clinical psychologist, counseling psychologist, school psychologist, and social psychologist. Psychology is the science of human behavior and deals with thinking, feelings, and actions. As a nonmedical science, psychology is vital to the mental health field, contributing both to the prevention of mental illness and to its diagnosis and to the care of patients.

Clinical psychologists assist in the diagnosis and care of persons with mental illness. Working in hospitals, clinics, and universities, these psychologists design and conduct research with physicians or other social scientists or they work alone. Clinical psychologists help the individual who is maladjusted to learn new and better habits of behavior.

Counseling psychologists try to get people to understand themselves so that they can deal sensibly with their problems, make worthwhile decisions, and use their abilities and opportunities to the best advantage. These psychologists prevent mental illness. Their services are needed in elementary and secondary schools, colleges and universities, industry, and mental health centers. Counseling psychologists are important in the rehabilitation of handicapped workers. These psychologists help the handicapped to readjust to their roles in families, communities, and jobs.

School psychologists are found in elementary and secondary schools and are concerned with the psychologic factors of the student. The gifted, handicapped, and disturbed students need the assistance of school psychologists who diagnose and plan corrective programs to help these students. These psychologists observe students in the classroom, study students' records, have conferences with teachers and parents, and administer and interpret psychologic tests. Often, school psychologists serve as consultants to school administrators and parents as to psychologic services within the schools.

Social psychologists are concerned with group reactions and behavior rather than with the individual. These psychologists try to find how our social attitudes develop, how individuals make up families and neighborhoods, and how individuals react upon each other in communities. Many of our problems affecting society become the concerns of social psychologists.

Psychometrists administer psychologic tests—often under the directions of psychologists. Questions on tests are carefully planned so that the responses of persons taking the tests will give clues to personality traits or psychologic difficulties. The psychometrist must be able to detect these clues and interpret them. Many types of tests are used by psychometrists. Some involve physical objects to be manipulated; others employ different kinds of testing devices.

Sociologists determine how such factors as a person's occupation, education, religion, family, community, ethnic customs, and prejudices affect his health. Sociology is the science of society, and this knowledge is extremely valuable to hospitals, industries, schools and colleges, and public health programs. Sociologists may specialize in a particular area of research such as society's attitudes toward health and illness.

They may be asked to find why there are unusual pressures on a hospital staff or how the social climate of a university affects students' attitudes. Some sociologists serve as consultants to industries; others work in federal health agencies, state and local health departments, hospitals, and mental health centers. Many sociologists teach in universities and professional schools, e.g., schools of nursing.

The health economist, through research, provides answers to the production, distribution, and use of health services to guarantee the greatest number of persons with the highest quality of medical care at the lowest cost. Private and group medical practice, rehabilitation services, hospitals, local and state health departments, and the United States Public Health Service employ health economists. As people can purchase more health services and these services grow, the health economist becomes increasingly important.

Social Worker

The social worker helps people with their jobs, families, financial problems, and daily tasks of living, particularly when their needs are related to illness and disability. The medical social worker helps the patient and his family handle problems that accompany severe illness or disability. If the problems are not resolved, the patient's recovery from illness or disability may be seriously delayed. When illness takes on crisis proportions for the patient and his family, the medical social worker tries to mobilize many community agencies to help them. For a patient living alone and convalescing from illness, the medical social worker may provide a home health aide.

The psychiatric social worker helps people who are mentally or emotionally disturbed and is a member of the mental health team. The psychiatric social worker obtains information about the patient when the patient enters a mental hospital or mental health clinic. The information is needed by the psychiatrist and includes medical history, family background and relationships, early childhood, education, work experiences, and social interests. The psychiatric social worker serves as a continuous contact between the family and the patient in the mental hospital. The nature of the patient's illness needs interpretation to the family, and the family must be prepared to accept the patient at recovery. When the patient returns to normal life, the psychiatric social worker is the link between the hospital and the community. Working with the medical social worker, the psychiatric social worker is employed by mental hospitals, mental health centers, child guidance clinics, federal hospitals providing psychiatric care, courts, rehabilitation organizations, and hospitals for the retarded and epileptic. Other persons in social work are the caseworker, groupworker, administrator, and assistants.

Other Health Specialists

Public health statisticians are employed by state and local health departments, the United States Public Health Service, federal agencies, industries, voluntary health agencies, medical schools, and scientific research institutions and as professors in schools of public health. The public health statistician is concerned with the incidence of disease, death and birth rates, life expectancy, marriage in all ethnic populations, and planning and evaluation of health services.

The biostatistician designs research projects to answer questions concerning health and disease. The biostatistician provides the research design, research techniques, and statistical testing devices. Since a substantial part of the processing and analysis of data is accomplished by electronic equipment, the biostatistician must be able to program and operate a computer.

The rehabilitation counselor tries to help the disabled to minimize his handicap by capitalizing on the disabled's skills and aptitudes so that the disabled can be employed. To do this, the rehabilitation counselor must know a great deal about the disabled person, administer many aptitude and psychologic tests, develop a vocational plan, provide job training in a job situation, and obtain a suitable job for the disabled. Rehabilitation counselors may specialize in working with the blind, mentally ill, retarded, paraplegics, and disabled who are socially disadvantaged. These counselors must know the employment situation and opportunities for the disabled. Thus, they divide their time between working with the disabled and with the community where they solicit jobs.

The radiologic health specialist seeks to control radiation, limit exposure to people, and minimize risks of radiation. Exposure to radiation must be balanced against the benefits of radiation. Unnecessary exposure must be eliminated. Radiation is used widely in medicine, dentistry, industry, research, and nucleur energy production. In agriculture, research scientists use radioactive substances to identify patterns of plant and animal growth. Pharmacists dispense radioactive drugs for diagnostic and therapeutic uses in medicine while veterinarians conduct studies of radiation effects on animals. Radiologic health specialists include the radiation monitor and the radiographer.

Food and drug inspectors and analysts are employed by the United States Department of Agriculture, the Food and Drug Administration, and state health departments. Food and drug laws have been enacted by the United States Congress and each state legislature.

To enforce federal food and drug laws, the federal government employs inspectors who are concerned with the purity and safety of foods and drugs and the effectiveness of drugs. When foods or drugs violate the law, they are seized in federal court actions. The inspectors provide protection before foods and drugs reach the customer. They work wherever the foods and drugs are—farms or manufacturing plants, processing plants, storage warehouses, transportation industry, food stores and restaurants, drug distribution centers, and stores selling drugs. They continuously check against accidental spoilage or contamination, collect samples of shipments, investigate complaints, and report evidence of law violations.

The analysts test the inspectors' samples more intensively than the inspectors do. Through laboratory work, the analysts check the purity of the inspectors' samples, do intensive research on the safety and effectiveness of products, detect spoilage and contamination, and test the composition of foods and drugs. In state health departments, the food and drug inspectors and analysts enforce state food and drug laws and work with federal food and drug inspectors and analysts. In most instances the food and drug industries cooperate with state and federal food and drug inspectors and analysts, since industry desires purity and safety of foods and drugs and effectiveness of drugs.

OTHER PROFESSIONAL WORKERS

Physicians and medical specialists, dentists and dental specialists, and professional nurses were included in Chapter 7. This section will focus upon the osteopath, podiatrist, physician's assistant, optometrist and optician, orthopotist, pharmacist, speech pathologist and audiologist, orthotist and prosthetist, mortician, veterinarian, and nurse-midwife.

Osteopathic Physician

The seven colleges of osteopathic medicine grant the degree of doctor of osteopathy (DO) after the candidate has a bachelor's degree, four years of osteopathic preparation, and a year of rotating internship. At least 80 teaching osteopathic hospitals have been approved by the American Osteopathic Association for intern training. Osteopathy stresses the importance of body mechanics to the health of the organism and emphasizes the use of manipulation to detect and correct faulty structure. Manipulative therapy, drugs, physical therapy, and other methods are used in treating illness and injury. Graduates of the osteopathic colleges are prepared as general practitioners. Many osteopaths extend their education into one or more of the following specialities: anesthesiology, internal medicine, dermatology, neurology and psychiatry, obstetrics and gynecology, ophthalmology, otorhinolaryngology, pathology, pediatrics, proctology, radiology, rehabilitation medicine, and surgery. All states have state licensing boards for osteopaths passing the state board examinations and educational qualifications. Osteopaths practice in the 310 osteopathic hospitals in the United States, as well as in other tax-supported hospitals.

Podiatrists

There are at least 8500 practicing doctors of podiatric medicine in the United States. A specialist in the care of the foot, the podiatrist diagnoses and treats diseases and deformities of the feet and tries to prevent these diseases and deformities. The podiatrist is continuously alert to signs of chronic health conditions such as arthritis, diabetes, and circulatory conditions, which manifest themselves in the foot. There are five accredited colleges of podiatric medicine in the United States. To become a podiatrist, the candiate must have at least two years of college work and four years of preparation in a college of podiatry. One-year and two-year residencies are available to students who want further experience. The degree of Doctor of Podiatric Medicine is granted upon completion of all podiatric college requirements. All states license podiatrists. A licensing examination is given by a state board of podiatry examiners or board of medical examiners, depending on the state. Podiatric assistants are among the emerging new health professionals.

Physician's Assistant

Routine duties requiring some medical skill become the responsibilities of the physician's assistant. Some medical schools offer preparation leading to the occupation of certified physician's assistant. The assistant may start the day by reporting to the hospital where he collects samples of patients' blood and other body contents requested by his physician-boss. He may administer injections ordered by the physician and get all materials to the proper laboratory for analysis. Then, he joins his physician-boss to whom he reports results of laboratory tests and other records pertinent to patients. With his physician-boss, he visits patients and receives instructions for further treatments or tests to be given within his professional capacity. In a small town he may give medical examinations, routine checkups, and laboratory tests. In many states no official guidelines have been established as to how much direct patient care can legally be given by a physician's assistant so that there is no risk of medical malpractice suits.

Optometrist and Optician

The doctor of optometry (OD) is educated and prepared to examine eyes to detect visual problems. The optometrist may prescribe eyeglasses, recommend other optical treatment, and refer the patient to an ophthalmologist if there is eye disease or injury. The optometrist fits lenses to frames suitable to the patient. The optometrist offers these additional services: prescribing and fitting contact lenses, discovering and solving children's vision problems, developing aids for the partially sighted such as telescopic lens for the older age groups, and vision training. All eleven American colleges of optometry require two to four years of preoptometric college study and four years of professional education for the degree of doctor of optometry. A comprehensive examination is given by state licensing boards of examiners of optometry.

The dispensing optician produces eyeglasses prescribed by an ophthalmologist. He grinds the lenses according to the prescription and patient's measurements, fits the lenses into the assembled frame, and adjusts the finished glasses. The mechanical work of grinding the surfaces of the lenses may be done by the optician or an optical technician. The dispensing optician instructs wearers of contact lenses how to insert, remove, and care for the contact lenses. Accurate measurements of the patient's cornea must be made by the optician for the patient who desires contact lenses. In states where the optician is licensed, he must be skillful in the technical work of lens grinding and fitting. These skills are needed to pass state licensing examinations. A beginner may start as an apprentice technician in a school of opticianry or a vocational school with courses in optical technology.

Orthoptist

The orthoptist teaches patients eye exercises that help misaligned eyes to work together and to see the same object with properly fused vision. The orthoptist works under the supervision of an ophthalmologist. Two to four years of college work precede the 15-month preparation in orthoptics. A certificate is issued to qualified students who pass an examination given by the American Orthoptic Council. Even though there are no legal requirements to obtain such certification, at least 95 percent of all medically trained orthoptists are certified.

Pharmacist

The primary responsibility of the pharmacist is to compound and dispense medicine as prescribed by a physician or other qualified practitioner. In addition, the pharmacist offers guidance in over-the-counter drugs or nonprescription medicine. The pharmacist must be fully acquainted with the physical and chemical properties of drugs, the effect of drugs on the human being, and the reaction to drugs in laboratory tests of blood and human tissues. The pharmacist must purchase and sell hundreds of health-related items and be proficient in the management of the pharmacy. The bachelor of science degree in pharmacy is completed in a five-year program of which three years must be in an accredited college of pharmacy. All states have strict laws about licensing and registration. Most states require internship or practical experience to obtain a license, in addition to passing an examination given by the state board of pharmacy. Most registered pharmacists are community pharmacists who are owners or managers of pharmacies. A newly licensed pharmacist may be an assistant to the community pharmacist. Pharmacists are employed in hospital pharmacies, nursing homes, extended care centers, clinics, laboratories of pharmaceutical companies, universities, research institutes, and professional schools such as medical schools and by the United States Public Health Service, all three branches of the Armed Forces, and the Veterans Administration.

Speech Pathologist and Audiologist

Since many children and adults have speech problems, the speech pathologist and audiologist help children and adults to communicate as nearly normally as possible. Some of the problems encountered by the speech pathologist and audiologist are lisping, cleft palate, impaired hearing, and talking difficulties from mental retardation, emotional disturbances, and cerebral palsy. The speech pathologist must have completed graduate study from a college with an acceptable department of speech pathology and audiology and have sufficient credits in speech and hearing to be certified by the National Association of Hearing and Speech Agencies. The audiologist will need graduate study in speech pathology and audiology. In addition to being employed by public schools, speech pathologists and audiologists are employed by federal, state, and local agencies providing services for crippled children; the Armed Forces; social agencies; medical centers; and clinics at colleges.

Orthotist and Prosthetist

The orthotist makes and fits orthopedic braces to support weakened body parts or to correct physical defects. The prosthetist makes and fits artificial limbs. Both work from a physician's prescription. They must obtain careful and accurate measurements from the patient, design a device to meet the needs of the patient, and construct the device from plastic, leather, steel, aluminum, or wood. The patient receives a preliminary fitting before the device is completed, whether it is a brace (orthosis) or an artificial limb (prosthesis). When the device is worn by the patient, it undergoes evaluation by the orthotist or prosthetist and by other rehabilitation specialists. From 1976 through 1979, a person wishing to be an orthotist and/or prosthetist must have an associate of arts degree in orthotics and/or prosthetics and have two years of clinical experience prior to graduation. By 1980, the person will have to possess a bachelor of science degree in orthotics and prosthetics. Also, the candidate must present recommendations from three orthopedic surgeons and pass the certification examination by the American Board for Certification in Orthotics and Prosthetics. Assistants and technicians certified by the board work under the direct supervision of the orthotist or prosthetist. The orthotic-prosthetic assistant is responsible for fabricating and fitting devices, and is closely involved in patient care. The orthotic-prosthtic technician does the fabrication of components and devices and has no direct patient-care activities.

Mortician

The funeral director or mortician prepares the dead human body for burial. The duties of the mortician involve his receiving the dead human body, embalming, restoring features of the deceased, transporting the deceased, providing the funeral service and burial, and complying with regulations of the burial permit, health codes, and cemetery ordinances. Embalming is the treatment of the dead body with antiseptics and preservatives to prevent putrefaction. Features of the deceased are restored so that the deceased is presentable at the funeral service. Morticians complete specialized professional education in mortuary science, followed by one to three years' apprenticeship. Most states require them to take the examination by a state board of morticians to obtain a license.

Veterinarian

The work of the veterinarian falls into three categories. First, he tries to have animals free from disease and teaches owners how to feed and care for the animals. Second, the veterinarian gives medical or surgical care to injured or ill animals. Third, he protects and promotes human health through inspection of foods of animal origin. Animal diseases that may be a possible threat to humans are brucellosis, rabies, and salmonellosis. At least six years of higher education are needed by the veterinarian—two years of preprofessional study at an agricultural college and four years of veterinary medicine, leading to the degree doctor of veterinary medicine (DVM). Most approved colleges of veterinary medicine prefer four years of preveterinary study leading to a bachelor's degree, followed by four years of veterinary medicine. A veterinarian must have a state license from the state in which he practices veterinary medicine. The license is granted after passing an examination given by the state board of veterinary medical examiners.

At least 60 percent of the veterinarians have private practices. Only a small number are employed by zoos and circuses. Eleven percent work in veterinary public health. Some with a private practice are rural veterinarians who take care of farm animals and teach the owners about diseases transmitted from animals to people. Others are urban veterinarians who treat household pets. Some rural and urban veterinarians combine private practice with part-time public health work such as inspection of poultry. Many times the new graduate veterinarian may be an assistant or junior partner to an established private practitioner.

Public health veterinarians may be employed by local and state health departments, the United States Public Health Service, the United States Department of Agriculture, the Food and Drug Administration, and by international groups such as the World Health Organization. In addition to his veterinary medicine education, the public veterinarian needs postgraduate study in an accredited school of public health. Veterinarians are in military veterinary medicine, research, and pharmaceutical companies. Some of the specialities in veterinary medicine, besides those already mentioned are:

Veterinarian, Laboratory Animal Care
Veterinary Anatomist
Veterinary Bacteriologist
Veterinary Livestock Inspector
Veterinary Meat Inspector
Veterinary Parsitologist
Veterinary Pharmacologist
Veterinary Physiologist
Veterinary Virologist
Veterinary Virus-Serum Inspector

The veterinarian's skills are needed in many fields of employment. In the practice of this profession, the veterinarian risks exposure to diseases and injury from animals.

Nurse–Midwife

A midwife is trained to give the necessary care to pregnant women during pregnancy, labor, and the postnatal period; to conduct normal deliveries of babies; and to care for the newly born infant. The midwife should be able to recognize the signs of abnormal conditions during pregnancy, to refer the pregnant woman with these conditions to a physician, and to carry out emergency services in the absence of medical care.

Nurse-midwives are taking the place of midwives of the past. Reasons for the upsurge in the preparation of nurse-midwives are (1) communities in which 25 to 45 percent of the births are not attended by any medical or nursing personnel, and (2) large city hospitals where the burden of obstetrics exceeds the capacity of the medical staff. The nurse-midwife provides obstetrical care for pregnant women who cannot afford medical and/or hospital care, for babies with handicaps or in environments not inducive to the best health care, for babies where hospitalization is not available and physicians are few in number, and for pregnant women who are ignorant of maternity care. Other duties include medical examination of the pregnant woman, pelvic examination and evaluation, and taking the Papanicolaou smear. If the labor is normal, the nurse-midwife will manage labor and perform the delivery. The nurse-midwife may give treatments, infusions, and medications in accordance with the physician's orders. She may perform postpartum examinations and instruct in methods of birth control. Nurse-midwife training may take place in a hospital, clinic, or nursing school. Graduate programs in midwife-teacher training may be two years in length or lead to a Master of Science degree in Nursing with a certificate in nurse-midwifery. A certification examination is given by the American College of Nurse-Midwives.

SANITARIANS AND ENGINEERS

Another group of health professions includes sanitarians, sanitary engineers, hospital engineers, biomedical engineers, and safety engineers.

Sanitarian

More than 8000 of the possible 10,000 professional sanitarians are employed by the federal, state, and local governments. Others work for processors of food products and institutions of higher learning. Sanitarians interpret and enforce city, state, and federal laws regarding sanitary standards in water supply, milk and food, garbage disposal, sewage or wastewater treatment, air pollution, housing maintenance, control of rodents and insects, and other environmental health measures. They supervise, inspect, and analyze reports of inspections made by other environmental health specialists, e.g., restaurant inspectors. If there is evidence of violations of public health regulations, they give evidence in court cases. In large city health departments, a sanitarian may specialize in a particular type of work such as food sanitarian. Some sanitarians in management positions are involved with planning and administering environmental health programs, advising governmental officials on environmental health problems, and drafting health laws. There are more than 5000 sanitary technicians and aides.

The preferred preparation of a sanitarian is a bachelor's degree in environmental health, followed by a year of on-the-job training under the supervision of an experienced sanitarian. After this trainee experience, the sanitarian may be promoted to minor supervisory responsibilities. At least 31 states have laws requiring the registration of sanitarians.

Sanitary Engineer

The design and operation of water purification processes, wastewater treatment, milk pasteurization plants, solid waste disposal as sanitary landfills, and other environmental health controls are the responsibilities of the sanitary engineer. Monitoring air pollution, noise, and radiologic hazards, as well as control of insects and rodents, are other responsibilities. Wastewater technology may include changes in engineering design to cope with detergents and remnants of household garbage grinders. Other environmental hazards for which new community engineering skills are needed are nuclear power plants, diversity of insecticides, increased number of disposable household items, and problems in occupational health.

Civil engineering with emphasis upon the sanitary sciences such as water purification is the main undergraduate preparation of the sanitary engineer. Graduate study in public health and sanitary engineering is encouraged. Most states require that sanitary engineers be registered or licensed. Specialty certification of sanitary engineers is provided by the American Academy of Sanitary Engineers. Other personnel working with sanitary engineers are the environmental technician and the environmental aide.

Chief Engineer of a Hospital

The hospital's chief engineer is responsible for the maintenance and upkeep of lighting, heating, plumbing, and elevator service; remodeling or expansion; and repair of mechanical, electrical, and building facilities. A variety of people with different skills are under his direction. He supervises these people, develops job specifications, makes assignments, checks that jobs are accomplished as they should be, and keeps personnel and supply records for his department. He must be familiar with mechanical, electrical, and building repairs. In large hospitals the hospital engineer has a college degree in mechanical or electrical engineering and considerable practical experience. Some of the maintenance workers supervised by the hospital's chief engineer are the operators of stationary boiler equipment, plumbers, electricians, carpenters, masons, painters, plasterers, and groundskeepers.

Bioengineer

Bioengineering is the preferred term to biomedical engineering, medical electronics, medical engineering, bioinstrumentation, biomedical instrumentation, and medical instrumentation. Bioengineering falls into the following areas: (1) development of new instruments in medical and surgical care or in research, (2) invention and perfection of devices to repair or compensate for parts of the human body not functioning properly or damaged, (3) adaptation of computer technology to health services and research; and (4) application of engineering theory and medical research in studies of the structure and functioning of the human body. Bioengineers have developed instruments, such as lasers, for use in medicine, surgery, radiology and other medical specialties. Such devices as external parts of the human body, electronically powered artificial limbs, heart-lung machine, electric defibrillator, heart pacemakers, and the artificial kidney machine have been developed to repair or compensate for parts of the human body not functioning properly or damaged. Bioengineers are adapting computers and electronic data processing machines to assist in compiling and analyzing health data. Bioengineers need preparation in engineering disciplines and in biology, biochemistry, physiology, and physics. Biomedical engineering technicians assist bioengineers and assemble, adapt, and maintain new instrumentation and devices.

Safety Engineer

Employed to minimize accident hazards and promote safe work habits, the safety engineer is vital in mines, industrial plants, and wherever industrial accidents may occur. This engineer tries to educate the worker in the proper use of equipment, prevent damage to equipment and materials, reduce heavy costs to personnel and insurance underwriters by eliminating accidents, and provide fire protection. The safety engineer investigates accidents, inspects working conditions and equipment, and finds the causes of accidents. He is expected to carry out extensive accident prevention programs, ensure compliance with industrial safety laws and standards, and develop safety rules. The safety engineer should have a bachelor's degree in engineering with emphasis upon safety education.

SERVICE SPECIALISTS, WORKERS, AND AIDES

Within this category are nutritionists, dietitians, the food service supervisor and workers, licensed practical nurses, home health aides and homemakers, and the executive housekeeper in a hospital.

Nutritionist

The nutritionist is concerned with teaching all ages about nutrition and helping special groups develop meal patterns related to their particular needs. These groups are the elderly, families on a limited income, foreign-born, and young mothers with their first babies. Nutritionists are employed by state and local health departments, the United States Public Health Service, local and state welfare programs, voluntary health agencies, universities and colleges, and international technical assistance programs. The communication of scientific knowledge about nutrition, organization and administration of nutrition surveys, and consultation with physicians, social workers, and public health nurses are some of the tasks of the nutritionist. Graduate study in nutrition is required in addition to health education.

Dietitian

There are four major areas of specialization in dietitics. First, the dietitian may be director of the department of dietetics in a hospital or a related health facility and be responsible for the food service to both patients and personnel. Second, the dietitian is a clinical or therapeutic dietitian who provides patients with nutritionally adequate meals and plans menus for patients with special needs. Third, the teaching dietitian conducts educational programs in dietetics for medical, nursing, and dental students; patients; and dietetic interns. Fourth, the research dietitian participates in planning and conducting nutrition research and is a member of the clinical research team. Most dietitians are employed in hospitals. However, dietitians are found in the military services, related health facilities, and university and school food services. Some dietitians are self-employed consultants working with physicians who have patients needing special nutrition guidance. A bachelor's degree with internship in dietetics, a master's degree, a coordinated program with practicum, or a bachelor's degree with traineeship is usually required by the American Dietetic Association (ADA). Graduate degrees are necessary for teaching dietitians and research dietitians. RD (Registered Dietitian) is given by the ADA to those dietitians who pass an examination and continue their education by earning a specified number of credits every five years.

Food Service Supervisors and Workers

Employed by elementary and secondary schools, junior colleges, colleges and universities, hospitals, and industrial organizations, food service supervisors are responsible for planning, preparing, and serving meals. The supervisors must train cooks, helpers, attendants and other workers. The supervisors plan daily menus, purchase food, provide adequate food storage, fulfill all sanitary measures, maintain cleanliness in food preparation and eating areas, comply with local health regulations, keep records, and handle finances. Supervisors are usually promoted from the ranks of the food workers. Food workers usually receive their training on the job and may specialize to be different cooks, vegetable or fruit helpers, and bakers. Other food workers are responsible for dishwashing and cleanliness of the kitchen and lunchroom.

Licensed Practical Nurse

The licensed practical nurse (LPN; LVN—licensed vocational nurse in California and Texas) is employed in hospitals, local health departments, rehabilitation agencies, nursing homes, physicians' offices, clinics, private homes, and special institutions such as a children's hospital. Many hospitals, junior colleges, and public vocational schools operate state-approved practical nursing schools. Most programs require high school graduation as a prerequisite to entering the licensed practical nurse training. Upon completion of a 12-month course, the practical nurse must pass a state board examination to obtain a license. Men are needed as practical nurses, especially in psychiatric and rehabilitation hospitals. Some LPN's prefer to work in a specific area of nursing such as medical-surgical, intensive care, psychiatric, and pediatric.

Home Health Aide and Homemaker

The home health aide may bathe and exercise the convalescent person, give the patient medicine prescribed, keep in contact with the patient's physician as to the patient's condition, assist in meal preparation, and feed the patient. The home health aide is involved with the physical and simple health needs of the convalescent, disabled, or homebound person.

The homemaker does the cleaning, shopping, and cooking and takes care of children while the mother is in the hospital or is ill. The homemaker is concerned with standard housekeeping services.

Executive Housekeeper in a Hospital

Housekeeping in a hospital includes general cleaning, laundry, window and wall washing, floor polishing, mending of bed linen and clothes, redecorating of rooms, and supervision of maids. The executive housekeeper promotes large-scale cleanliness, establishes standards and work methods, prepares work schedules, hires and trains all housekeeping personnel, and inspects the work of all housekeeping personnel. Many executive housekeepers have a college degree in institutional management or home economics. Some of the housekeeping personnel are porters, maids, linen-room attendants, and clothes-room workers. Even though the executive housekeeper supervises the laundry maintained by the hospital, many large hospitals have a laundry manager who supervises the washing and finishing of laundry and directs the training of new laundry workers. In some hospitals, the laundry manager prepares sterile packs for use in surgery, delivery rooms, and nurseries.

TECHNOLOGISTS, TECHNICIANS, THERAPISTS, HYGIENISTS, AND ASSISTANTS

These health careers include medical technologists and related occupations: medical laboratory technician, certified laboratory assistant, cytotechnologist, histologic technician, blood bank technologist, electrocardiograph technician, electroencephalograph technologist, and nuclear medicine technologist and technician. Other technologists will be food technologists and radiologic technologists. The therapists will include physical therapists and assistants, occupational therapists and assistants, corrective therapists, educational therapists, manual arts therapists, music therapists, recreational therapists, and inhalation therapists. Finally, there are industrial hygienists, dental hygienists, dental assistants, dental laboratory technicians, and medical assistants.

Medical Technologist

Laboratory examinations of body fluids and tissues assist the physician in his diagnosis of the patient. These examinations are performed by medical technologists and technicians. The use of the electrocardiogram by an electrocardiograph technician is another of the related occupations of medical technology.

Some of the tests performed by the medical technologists are:

1. Testing for antibodies and other disease-fighting substances in the blood
2. Doing blood tests to detect illnesses of the blood such as leukemia, hemophilia, mononucleosis, and anemia, or a chronic health condition such as diabetes
3. Analyzing urine for evidence of diabetes, nephritis, infection of the bladder, cancer of the bladder
4. Matching blood samples of the donor and recipient in blood transfusions
5. Culturing bacteria found in the patient's sputum, blood, feces, or discharge from a sore or wound
6. Identifying parasites, such as pinworms
7. Testing for the presence or absence of different chemicals in the blood and other body tissues

The medical technologist must have three years in college plus one year of clinical education in medical technology. The clinical education lasts 12 months. Graduates can receive certification by passing an examination of either the Registry of Medical Technologists of the American Society of Clinical Pathologists or the American Medical Technologists' registry and one year of approved laboratory experience.

The medical laboratory technician does the routine laboratory tests under the supervision of the medical technologist. An associate degree from an accredited junior or community college and clinical experience in an approved laboratory are required. Certification as a medical laboratory technician may be had from the Registry of Medical Technologists and the American Medical Technologists' registry, provided the technician has a two-year work-school experience.

The certified laboratory assistant works under the supervision of a medical technologist in routine laboratory procedures such as urinalysis. A 12-month program in a school approved by the American Medical Association is required for certification as a laboratory assistant. Some hospital laboratory schools are accredited to provide high school graduates with one year of training in routine laboratory work. Certification may be obtained.

The cytotechnologist examines changes in body cells and works under the supervision of a pathologist. The cytotechnologist screens slides of cell samplings and uses special dyes to detect possible diseases or cancer. Two years of college work, six months' study in an approved school of cytotechnology, and six months' experience in an acceptable cytology laboratory are required. The cytotechnologist may take a certifying examination given by the Registry of Medical Technologists.

The histologic technician cuts and stains body tissues so that these tissues can be examined by the pathologist. These tissues are examined particularly for malignant cells. A year of supervised training in histologic technique is required. An examination for certification is given by the Registry of Medical Technologists.

The Blood bank technologist collects blood from donors, processes it, classifies it, and stores it either as whole blood or as plasma. These technologists work in blood bank centers, hospitals, and clinics. As certified medical technologists, these technologists have had another year of education in a blood bank school approved by the American Association of Blood Banks. An examination for certification is given by the Registry of Medical Technologists.

The electrocardiograph technician uses the ECG or EKG machine which records heart actions, helps to diagnose heart disease, and records progress of patients with heart conditions. This technician may work in a clinic, hospital, or rehabilitation center. Three to six months of on-the-job training under the supervision of an experienced technician or cardiologist is required. The technician must know not only how to operate the machine but also how to get the correct machine tracing from the patient.

The electroencephalograph technician operates the EEG which records brain waves and indicates whether such conditions as a brain tumor, epilepsy, or stroke are present or have occurred. The brain wave tracings are interpreted by a neurologist. This technologist must have a fundamental understanding of not only the EEG but also the health conditions encountered in brain activity during sleep and wakefulness. Most training of these technicians is of the on-the-job type combined with study of the nervous system, basic instrumentation, diseases of the brain, and care of the patient. A one-year training period consisting of six months of basic preparation and six months of supervised practice is preferred. A registered EEG technologist must pass an examination given by the American Board of Registration of EEG Technologists.

The nuclear medical technologist uses radioactive isotopes to diagnose disease and is mainly involved in laboratory work. This technologist injects or inserts the isotopes into the circulatory system, tissue, or organ. Since few opportunities are available to prepare for this job, most nuclear medical technologists are certified medical technologists who gained experience in nuclear medicine laboratories or who had four years of college work in science and two years of experience in nuclear medicine laboratories. Nuclear medical technicians are involved with routine tasks in this field. These technologists and technicians are employed in hospitals with departments of nuclear medicine, veterans' hospitals, and nuclear medicine laboratories.

Food Technologist

The food technologist applies science and engineering to the production, processing, packaging, distribution, prepartion, evaluation, and utilization of foods. This technologist solves problems which occur with the development of products, processes, or equipment; changes in the physical condition of any food undergoing industrial processing; selection of raw materials; or changes in the nutritional values of foods. Other tasks include preventing food spoilage and improving preservatives used in foods, testing raw materials and finished products, and developing new sources of natural and synthetic foods. Some colleges have a separate department of food technology, some have a program leading to a bachelor's degree, and others offer graduate study in food technology. Nutrition, science, and engineering should be the main programs of study.

Radiologic Technologist

X-rays reveal injuries to bones, diseases of internal organs, and abnormalities within an organ or tissues. X-rays can be used in treatment of certain diseases. Diagnostic X-ray technology and radiation therapy technology are two of the fields of radiologic technology. The diagnostic X-ray technologist operates X-ray equipment and makes radiographs (on X-ray film) of various parts of the human body. The radiation therapy technologist operates X-ray therapy machines and prepares, administers, and measures radioactive isotopes as prescribed by the radiologist.

These technicians need a year or two of college work with emphasis on physics and chemistry and courses in radiologic technology over a period of 24 months. Some colleges offer a bachelor of science degree in X-ray technology. The technologist graduated from a school or college approved by the American Medical Association can receive certification from the American Registry of Radiologic Technologists.

Physical Therapist

Working under the direction of physicians, the physical therapist rehabilitates people with injuries, diseases, and chronic health conditions in muscles, joints, bones, or nerves. Exercise, massage, and applications of heat, light, electricity, and water are used. Persons having arthritis, amputations, fractures, nerve injuries, multiple sclerosis, muscular dystrophy, cerebral palsy, and other disabling conditions use the services of physical therapists. Physical therapists teach the families of the disabled how to carry on physical therapy at home and how to care for and use braces or prosthetic appliances.

There are three basic plans of education for physical therapy: four-year Bachelor of Science degree in physical therapy; 12 months certificate courses for students with a bachelor's degree; and graduate study leading to a Master of Science degree in physical therapy. New graduates profit by having a year of experience under the supervision of experienced physical therapists, in addition to supervised clinical practice. Registration is required in 49 states, the District of Columbia, and Puerto Rico. The American Physical Therapy Association has a list of state boards of physical therapy examiners.

Employment is available in hospitals, specialized institutions such as those for veterans, rehabilitation centers, large industrial firms, schools for crippled children, Armed Forces, hospitals of the United States Public Health Service, and teaching and research. Many physical therapists establish their own clinics to which physicians refer patients.

The physical therapy assistant is a graduate of a two-year college with an associate degree in physical therapy. This assistant is a skilled worker who assists the physical therapist in patient treatment.

The physical therapy aide receives training on the job. This aide performs designated routine tasks related to physical therapy.

Occupational Therapist

To help patients with physical and emotional disabilities adjust to everyday living and other occupations, the occupational therapist uses various selected activities. Particularly, this therapist helps the handicapped to adjust to a possible change in occupation. The majority of occupational therapists are employed by hospitals. Others are needed in the specialized care of the aged or of persons with mental illness, cerebral palsy, or heart disease. Community health centers, rehabilitation agencies, veterans' and other federal hospitals, and nursing homes employ occupational therapists. A bachelor of science degree with emphasis in occupational therapy and a clinical training period are required. A national registration examination is conducted by the American Occupational Therapy Association.

The occupational therapy assistant works under the supervision of an occupational therapist. The assistant prepares and distributes materials and supplies, maintains tools and equipment, instructs patients in manual and creative arts, and reports to and consults with the occupational therapist regarding the patient's progress. Accredited junior or community colleges offer a two-year associate degree program, an accredited educational institution offers a one-year program or a hospital provides a 20- to 25-week program. Certification is available from the American Occupational Therapy Association.

Specialized Rehabilitation Services

Among personnel in specialized rehabilitation services are the corrective therapist, educational therapist, manual arts therapist, music therapist, recreational therapist, and industrial therapist. These persons work to restore the physically or emotionally handicapped to normal or near normal functioning.

The corrective therapist or therapist in adapted physical education may teach exercise routines to wheelchair patients, teach orthopedically handicapped to walk and move around, guide the blind in independent movement, train patients to use artificial limbs and braces, and provide exercise for the mentally ill and mentally retarded. Exercise routines for the physically handicapped are aimed to develop strength, dexterity, and coordination of muscles.

The educational therapist works with patients who because of their disability are detached from normal life, withdrawn, depressed, or agitated. The therapist attempts to stimulate interest, confidence, and self-esteem; overcome abnormal emotions; and restore a connection with other people. Hospitals, the Veterans Administration, and private and state-supported institutions employ educational therapists.

The manual arts therapist uses work activities of an agricultural and industrial nature in actual work situations to assist patients in their recovery. The activities serve to retrain the patient in a skill or trade or, if the disability makes this impossible, to train the patient in a new skill or trade. The main purpose is to engage the patient in an activity that gives him a sense of achievement and confidence, absorbs him, and motivates the patient to try to recover from his illness or injury.

The music therapist devises such programs as group singing, music appreciation, instrumental instruction, and simple orchestration for the disabled, physically or mentally. Psychiatric hospitals employ music therapists who plan music programs to achieve aims prescribed by the psychiatrist. Mental health teams at outpatient clinics as well as institutions with children who are mentally retarded, crippled, or blind, have music therapists.

The recreational therapist uses recreation in the rehabilitation of persons who are ill, physically disabled, or mentally retarded. The therapeutic recreation may be provided in a community setting, hospital, or other health facility. Sports, drama, or arts and crafts are used. The therapist often supervises volunteer assistants.

The industrial therapist places patients in a realistic work environment in a paying job. Some of the jobs are grounds and building maintenance, painting, gardening, and laundry or kitchen work. The therapist chooses work that will have the greatest therapeutic value for the patient and will prepare the patient for employment outside.

Inhalation Therapist

The inhalation therapist receives a prescription from the physician as to the type of therapy, medication, and dosage needed by the patient. The therapist must set up and operate therapeutic gas and mist inhalation equipment such as tanks, respirators, masks, catheters, cannulas, and incubators. The therapist determines the most suitable method of administering the inhalant, inserts the cannula or catheter, takes necessary precautions, and makes modifications to fit the physician's prescription. The therapist has to explain the inhalation treatment to the patient. This therapist operates the Intermittent-Positive-Pressure-Breathing machine. While treatment is in progress, the patient's general condition is observed. The therapist may conduct pulmonary function tests of various types such as blood gas analysis. Other functions include keeping equipment clean, sterile, and in good working condition; ordering repairs and new equipment; maintaining adequate supplies of oxygen and other gases; and conducting on-the-job instruction in inhalation therapy. A bachelor's degree and more than a year of on-the-job training under strict supervision are required. To become registered by the American Registry of Inhalation Therapists, the candidate must satisfactorily complete the educational and experience requirements and pass oral and written examinations.

Industrial Hygienist

The industrial hygienist has three functions: to detect industrial hazards, evaluate the seriousness of the hazards; and eliminate or control the hazards. At times drastic changes need to be made due to unsafe conditions within an industrial plant. Equipment may need to be modified or replaced, less toxic materials substituted for toxic ones, or operations shut down. Some of the industrial conditions affecting the worker are noise, fungi, radiation, poor lighting, vibration, fatigue, and discomfort. Besides working in industry, the hygienist is employed by transportation companies, public utilities, state and local health departments, mining companies, insurance companies, and the federal government. A college degree with a major in engineering is the basic educational requirement. A master's degree in safety education, engineering, or one of the physical sciences is advisable.

Dental Hygienist

The main tasks of the dental hygienist are cleaning teeth, providing diagnostic aids for the dentist, instructing in dental health education, applying fluorides to the teeth, and educating patients in nutrition as related to the teeth. The dental hygienist works under the supervision of a licensed dentist. Most dental hygienists are employed in private dentists' offices. Others work in public schools, state and local health departments' clinics, hospitals, industries, and rehabilitation centers. A bachelor's degree with a major in dental hygiene is usually required. Also, a state board dental hygiene licensing examination must be passed to practice dental hygiene in the state where the hygienist resides. The examination given by the National Board of Dental Hygiene may be substituted for the written test of the state board examination. Some community colleges offer a two-year program leading to a certificate or associate degree in dental hygiene.

Dental Assistant and Laboratory Technician

One or more dental assistants may be found in the dentist's office. The assistant prepares patients for examination and treatment, sterilizes instruments, assists the dentist while the patient is undergoing treatment, prepares dental materials such as fillings, and assists the dentist in taking X-rays. In addition, the assistant makes appointments and handles business transactions. Accredited dental assistant courses are offered in dental schools, community or junior colleges, and technical institutes. Certification is available from the Certifying Board of the American Dental Assistants' Association by completing an examination of written and clinical tests.

The dental laboratory technician makes and repairs dentures, crowns, bridges, and inlays under the prescription of a licensed dentist. The technician's skills complement those of the dentist, since the technician is designing and developing new equipment. Most dental laboratory technicians learn their skills through on-the-job training as an apprentice in a dental laboratory. Most dental laboratory technicians are employed by commercial dental laboratories.

Medical Assistant

Some of the functions of the medical assistant in the physician's office are to assist the physician when giving some medical examinations, obtain health histories from patients, assist the physician in emergency situations, order medical supplies, arrange hospital admissions, and complete medical reports and insurance forms. In addition, the medical assistant may serve as a receptionist, secretary, or administrative aide. Most junior or community colleges offer a two-year associate degree program for medical assistants. Certification can be obtained from the American Association of Medical Assistants if the college providing the preparation is approved by the American Medical Association.

REFERENCES

1. Office of the Federal Register, National Archives, and Records Service. General Services Administration: United States Government Manual, 1973/74. Washington, D.C., U.S. Government Printing Office, 1973, pp. 225-232.
2. Ibid., p. 224.
3. Haag, J. H.: School Health Program, 3rd Edition. Philadelphia, Lea & Febiger, 1972, p. 161.
4. Ibid., pp. 219-223.

SUPPLEMENTAL READINGS

American Medical Association: Horizons Unlimited: Career Opportunities in Medicine and Allied Fields. Chicago, The Association, 1966.
Fry, H. G.: Education and Manpower for Community Health. Pittsburgh, University of Pittsburgh Press, 1967.
Health Services and Mental Health Administration: Training the Auxiliary Health Worker. Health Service Publication 1817. Washington, D.C., U.S. Government Printing Office, 1968.
Lecht, L.: Manpower Needs for National Goals in the 1970s. New York, Frederick A. Praeger, Inc., 1969.
Lee, E. E.: Careers in the Health Field. New York, Julian Messner, Inc., 1972.
National Center for Statistics, U. S. Public Health Service: Health Resource Statistics. Washington, D.C., U.S. Government Printing Office, yearly.
National Commission on Community Health Services: Health Manpower Action to Meet Community Needs. Washington, D.C., Public Affairs Press, 1967.
Odgers, R., and Wenberg, B. G.: Introduction to Health Professions. St. Louis, C. V. Mosby Company, 1972.
Wilson, R. N.: Community Structure and Health Action: A Report on Process Analysis. Washington, D.C., Public Affairs Press, 1968.
Yahraes, H.: What's in Your Future—A Career in Health? #281. New York, Public Affairs Committee, 1968.

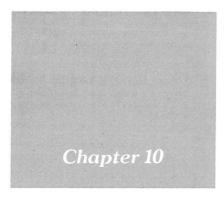

Chapter 10

CONSUMER PROTECTION AGENCIES

HUGE and complex problems face the consumer of health products and services. In many cases the consumer has not bothered to inform himself about the products and services he purchases. In addition, the consumer is not aware of the consumer agencies to assist him.

Consumers have been slow in organizing through citizen action. Consumers Union has less than 300,000 members and The Consumer Federation of America has limited lobby power compared with agricultural, business, and labor groups.

Today's consumer consciousness represents a deep-rooted public desire for a new-value system in the marketplace. Governmental agencies have begun to require the manufacturer to substantiate advertising claims for his products. Legislators are aware of consumer consciousness and are eager to support new agencies for consumer protection. Since the 18 to 24 age group is increasing rapidly, this age group may reach 29.6 million and be the most consumer conscious of any age group.

GOVERNMENTAL AGENCIES

Some of the federal departments and agencies that protect the consumer are the Department of Agriculture, Office of Consumer Affairs, Food and Drug Administration, and other agencies in the Public Health Service, Federal Trade Commission, Department of Labor, Social Security Administration, and Postal Service.

Department of Agriculture

In the Marketing and Consumer Services section of the Department of Agriculture, there is the Agricultural Marketing Services

(AMS). This service has developed standards for grades such as U.S. Grade A for most important farm commodities. Also, this service administers an inspection program of domestic, imported, and exported egg products; sets standards; and supervises processing of egg products. The Agricultural Marketing Service regulates certain business practices of dealers of farm commodities, insures truth in certain labels, covers the licensing, bonding, and examination of warehouses, and protects farmers' rights to organize cooperatives. The AMS helps to establish and maintain orderly marketing conditions for milk, fruits, vegetables, tobacco, nuts, and hops. Marketing regulatory programs are found in AMS, along with other programs to encourage diversion of surplus commodities from normal channels of trade to new markets.

The Animal and Plant Health Inspection Service conducts programs to protect the wholesomeness of meat and poultry products and to improve animal and plant health. It administers federal laws pertaining to animal and plant health and quarantine, meat and poultry inspection, and eradication of plant pests and diseases. Inspection is made of all meat, poultry, and related products processed by plants shipping in interstate and foreign commerce. Veterinary services officials determine the existence and extent of outbreaks of communicable diseases and pests affecting livestock and poultry. They work with state officials in disease control and inspect imported animals at ports of entry.

The Food and Nutrition Service administers the Food Stamp Program, Food Distribution Program, and Child Nutrition Programs. In the Food Distribution Program, food is given to needy persons by direct distribution. Child Nutrition Programs include the National School Lunch Program, School Breakfast Program, Special Food Service Program for Children (year-round program available to public and nonprofit private institutions providing day care for children from low-income areas), Equipment Program, and Special Milk Program for Children.

Packers and Stockyards Administration has as its principal objective to assist in the maintenance of free competitive practices in marketing of livestock, meat, poultry, and meat and poultry products.

The Statistical Reporting Service prepares estimates and reports of production, supply, price, and other items of agricultural economy.

The Commodity Exchange Authority maintains fair and honest trading practices and competitive pricing on commodity exchanges. The trading regulations prevent price manipulation and dissemination of false and misleading crop and market information. In addition, the regulations protect market users against fraud, cheating, and abusive practices in transactions. This agency has the responsibility for investigations of trading and market operations and providing information to the public on trading and marketing.

The Commodity Exchange Commission was established to initiate complaints, conduct hearings, and issue cease and desist or suspension orders for violations of the establishing act by the commodity exchange.

Consumer Affairs

Office of the Secretary of the Department of Health, Education, and Welfare administers the Office of Consumer Affairs. This Office was created to advise the President on all matters related to consumer interest.

The Consumer Product Safety Commission is an independent federal regulatory agency for the purpose of establishing mandatory safety standards to reduce the risk of injury to consumers from consumer products.

The Consumer Product Information Program is found in the General Services Administration and has two functions. It encourages Federal agencies to develop and release relevant and useful consumer information and to make the public aware of this information.

The National Business Council for Consumer Affairs Staff is in the Department of Commerce and advises the President and government agencies, through the Secretary of Commerce, in the area of consumer affairs and assists in voluntary programs for industry action to anticipate and resolve consumer problems.

In the Department of Justice, there is an Antitrust Division which has a Consumer Affairs Section. It is responsible for civil and criminal proceedings in cases referred to the Department of Justice by other agencies, such as the Federal Trade Commission.

Food and Drug Administration

In the Department of Health, Education, and Welfare is the Public Health Service which has five agencies, one being the Food and Drug Administration. Divisions of the FDA include the Bureau of Biologics, Bureau of Drugs, Bureau of Foods, Bureau of Radiological Health, Bureau of Veterinary Medicine, National Center for Toxicological Research, and Executive Director of Regional Operations. The activities of the FDA protect the health of Americans against impure and unsafe foods, drugs, and cosmetics, and other potential hazards.

The Bureau of Biologics administers regulations of biological products shipped in interstate and foreign commerce. These regulations pertain to manufacturers' facilities, testing of released products, approval for licenses to manufacture biological products, research related to new and old biological products, and evaluation of claims of new drugs.

The Bureau of Drugs develops standards and conducts research with respect to the safety, reliability, and efficacy of drugs. The Bureau evaluates new drug applications and claims for investigational drugs. It conducts clinical studies and operates an adverse drug reaction reporting system. The Bureau develops regulations, model codes, and other standards affecting the drug industry. It directs the antibiotic and insulin certification program. False labeling of drugs and adverse reactions to drugs found by consumers should be brought to the attention of this Bureau.

The Bureau of Foods conducts research and develops standards on the quality, nutrition, composition, and safety of foods, food additives, colors, and cosmetics. It conducts research to improve the detection and prevention of contamination conveyed by foods, cosmetics, and dyes. It develops regulations for food standards to permit the safe use of color and food additives. The Bureau collects and interprets data on food additives and nutrition.

The Bureau of Radiological Health conducts programs to reduce the exposure of man to hazardous radiation. These programs include safe limits of radiation exposure, health effects of radiation exposure, and radiation control to protect the public's health and safety. The Bureau sets standards to control the emission of radiation from electronic products.

The Bureau of Veterinary Medicine develops programs related to the efficacy and safety of veterinary preparations and devices. It evaluates proposed veterinary preparations and FDA compliance programs affecting veterinary drugs and other veterinary medical items.

The National Center for Toxicological Research conducts research programs to study the biological effects of toxic chemical substances in man's environment. It is concerned with the health effects of long-term low-level exposure to chemical intoxicants. The National Center develops methods and test protocols for evaluation of the safety of chemical toxicants and data to facilitate the extension of toxicological data from laboratory animals to man.[1]

In 1952, the first Consumer Specialists were hired by the FDA on a part-time basis. In 1964 each District was assigned a full-time specialist as part of the Consumer Education Program. These specialists are located in all of the Agency's districts. They maintain close and continuing touch with those people for whom the FDA's laws were written to protect; find the concerns consumers have about specific products; and discover problems of health, safety, and economic well-being of consumers. They handle consumer complaints and inquiries at the field level. They conduct countless formal and informal activities to educate the public. These specialists keep their eyes and ears open for specific types of consumer complaints or problems. They provide the FDA educational information for radio and television stations, newspapers, and other media. They are responsible for answering questions of local consumers concerning products that the FDA regulates. The consumer specialists may acquaint the public with the FDA's functions.[2]

Health Resources Administration

The Health Resources Administration is another agency of the Public Health Service and provides national leadership related to the requirements for and the distribution of health resources, including manpower training. The major components are Bureau of Health Manpower Education, Comprehensive Health Planning Service, Health Maintenance Organization Service, and National Center for Health Services Research and Development. The Bureau of Health Manpower Education administers programs to increase the effectiveness, supply, and availability of health manpower. The Comprehensive Health Planning Service considers the whole range of health concerns, with attention devoted to personnel, environmental, and mental health needs, problems, and programs. The Health Maintenance Organization Service aids the development of organized systems of health care for delivery of comprehensive services on a prepaid capitation basis. This Service maintains a national clearinghouse for information about HMO's. The National Center for Health Services and Development conducts and supports research and development focused at major health care problems of rising costs, inadequate access, and indefinite quality. The Center's major efforts include developing prototype health services systems, alternatives to hospital care, and cost-effective technology and evaluating new types of health service manpower.

Health Services Administration

Within the Public Health Service, the Health Services Administration provides professional leadership in the delivery of health services. The major components are Community Health Service, Federal Health Programs Service, Indian Health Services, Maternal and Child Health Service, and National Center for Family Planning Services. The Community Health Service acts as professional adviser to the Social Security Administration concerning medical standards and policies and procedures for the Medicare program and provides training for State agency personnel evaluating health facilities. Also, it organizes services for groups with special needs, residents of sparsely populated areas, and migrant farmworkers.

Center for Disease Control

In addition to the Health Services Administration of the United States Public Health Service, there is the Center for Disease Control. Among its many functions, the Center (1) provides consultation in upgrading the performance of clinical laboratories and evaluates and licenses clinical laboratories in interstate commerce and (2) offers policy guidance and administrative management of the National Institute of Occupational Safety and Health. This Institute develops and establishes recommended occupational safety and health standards.

National Institutes of Health

The National Institutes of Health of the United States Public Health Service conduct and support biomedical research into the causes, prevention, and cure of diseases and communicate biomedical information. The major components of the National Institutes of Health are the National Cancer Institute; National Heart and Lung Institute; National Institute of Mental Health; National Library of Medicine; National Institute of Arthritis, Metabolism, and Digestive Diseases; National Institute of Allergy and Infectious Diseases; National Institute of Child Health and Human Development; National Institute of Dental Research; National Institute of Environmental Health Sciences; National Institute of General Medical Sciences; Ntional Institute of Neurological Diseases and Stroke; and National Eye Institute.

Federal Trade Commission

The Federal Trade Commission, which was organized in 1915 as an independent administrative agency, prohibits in commerce "unfair methods of competition" and "unfair or deceptive acts or practices." Its main focus is to prevent through cease-and-desist orders and other means those practices condemned by the laws regulating federal trade. The Commission has ten principal functions. Among its functions for consumer protection, it promotes free and fair competition in interstate commerce. Second, the Commission prevents the dissemination of false or deceptive advertisements of food, drugs, cosmetics, and therapeutic devices. Third, it prevents discriminations in price, exclusive-dealing, and corporate mergers when such practices may lessen competition or tend toward monopoly and discrimination among competing customers. Fourth, it enforces truthful labeling of textile and fur products. Fifth, the Commission regulates packaging and labeling of certain consumer products so as to prevent consumer deception. Sixth, it protects consumers against the circulation of inaccurate credit reports and insures that consumer reporting agencies exercise their responsibilities in a fair and equitable manner. In Chapter 5, the legal case work of the Commission was described.

Department of Labor

Within the Employment Standards Administration of the Department of Labor is the Office of Workmen's Compensation Program. This Office administers federal workmen's compensation laws and related programs in connection with job-related injuries for persons in covered private employment. In addition, this Office administers such laws as the black lung portion of the Coal Mine Health and Safety Act extending benefits to coal miners afflicted with pneumoconiosis and their survivors.

The Assistant Secretary for Occupational Safety and Health Administration has the responsibility for occupational safety and health activities. Among these activities are the development of occupational safety and health standards, issuance of regulations, and investigations to determine the status of compliance with standards and regulations.

Social Security Administration

Medicare, Medicaid, and other health insurance are under the control of the Social Security Administration (SSA). Also, the SSA administers the black lung benefit provisions of the Coal Mine Health and Safety Act of 1969. The Administration has four program bureaus: Retirement and Survivors Insurance, Disability Insurance, Health Insurance, and Supplemental Security Income for the Aged, Blind, and Disabled. The Bureau of Retirement and Survivors Insurance provides direction for administration of retirement and survivors insurance programs and for procedures common to all social security programs. The Bureau of Disability Insurance reviews and authorizes the disability and black lung benefit claims. In addition, this Bureau works with the Social and Rehabilitation Service concerning the disability beneficiary rehabilitation program. The Bureau of Health Insurance develops principles for reimbursing hospitals, extended care facilities, and home health agencies for their costs and criteria for determining reasonable charges by physicians and for related medical services. The Bureau of Supplemental Security Income for the Aged, Blind, and Disabled develops and issues policies, procedures, and interpretations to the supplemental security income administration throughout the SSA.

Postal Service

Postal Service is an enormous service organization that commenced operations in July, 1971. They are five regional organizations to which the 85 districts report. The districts are divided into 321 sectional Center Manager Areas which have nearly 32,000 post offices throughout the United States.

The Postal Service protects the mails, postal funds, and property through its Inspection Service. Health quackery items sold or distributed by mail are investigated by the Postal Service. Postal Fraud statutes prohibit the use of the mails to obtain money or property by means of false or fraudulent pretenses or promises. These statutes permit the Postal Service to refuse delivery of mail to the promoter of the quack item. In addition, this Inspection Service apprehends those persons who violate the postal laws and investigates internal conditions and needs which may affect its effectiveness.

There is a Consumer Advocate, a postal ombudsman. This Advocate represents the interests of the individual mail customer by bringing complaints and suggestions to the top management of the Postal Service and solving the problems of consumers.

Other Federal Governmental Agencies

The Department of Health, Education, and Welfare has the Social and Rehabilitation Service with four component agencies. Medical Services Administration provides medical services to the needy and the medically needy. It works with the other federal agencies, state and local health organizations to extend the scope and quality of medical care to the needy. It develops medical care management and information systems, methods, and procedures.

The Federal Communications Commission regulates radio and television broadcasting, telephone, telegraph and cable television operation, two-way radio and radio operators, and satellite communication. It issues authorization for construction permits, licenses, modifications, renewals, assignments, and transfers in these services. It oversees compliance with the fairness doctrine and fair competition. The investigative and enforcement work of the Commission is done by its field staff. There are 30 field offices and 19 monitoring stations, in addition to a mobile network. The field staff are the "eyes and ears" of the Commission in detecting violations and enforcing rules and regulations.

Other federal agencies interested in consumer affairs are the Department of Commerce through its Domestic and International Business Administration, Interstate Commerce Commission, Small Business Administration, Extension Service of the Department of Agriculture, and Department of Housing and Urban Development.[3]

State and Local Agencies

Most state health departments have divisions or bureaus of food and drugs, health facilities construction, milk and dairy products (inspection), medical care administrative services, hospital licensing, nursing and convalescent homes (inspection and licensing), veterinary public health (meat and poultry inspection), product safety, occupational safety, radiation control, local health services, public health nursing, and special health services. The food and drug divisions have many tasks, among which may be investigating quick cures and quack products, food fads, mechanical quack items, coloring agents in food, labeling of foods and drugs, food additives, and quality of foods and drugs and measuring insecticide residues in food. Veterinary public health controls animal diseases transmissible to man, whether rabies or trichinosis. The public health veterinarians receive, tabulate, and prepare veterinary morbidity reports and serve as consultants to the food and drug personnel. The hospital licensing division is responsible for surveying, registering, and licensing of hospitals. It provides fire prevention, safety, and sanitation inspections of the hospital's physical plant and operations. Many of state health department's consumer protection interests may be similar to those of federal agencies.

Most states have a Department of Agriculture, Department of Labor, Department of Commerce, and Department of Education. These state departments have divisions or bureaus with consumer interests.

Offices of Consumer Affairs are not uncommon in state and local governments. At least 20 States have consumer protection agencies. The rising surge of consumer complaints on health quackery, food faddism, cults, mail-order health insurance, quacks posing as medical doctors, and poorly delivered health care have necessitated these consumer offices. Directors of these state and local consumer protection agencies give these tips to consumers:

1. Place complaint in writing.
2. Aim high when complaining. (A company president has better hearing than a sales clerk.)
3. Buy products, not packages. (The cover can hide the product.)
4. Check bills carefully.
5. Read the small print.
6. Demand written estimates for work.
7. Use credit to buy wisely.
8. Pay for the product you really want, not some "bargain" that is inferior in quality.
9. Be informed as to how local, state, and federal lawmakers protect consumers.
10. Shop in different places and compare prices.
11. Get full information about products.
12. Support independent consumer protection agencies in your locality and state.

The most important thing every consumer can do is to get together with another consumer—and another, and another—until their voices and purchasing decisions are heard in the marketplace.

NONGOVERNMENTAL AGENCIES

Some of the nongovernmental agencies are Consumer Federation of America, Consumers Union, Better Business Bureaus, American Medical Association, American Dental Association, American Dietetic Association, and National Dairy Council. The work of Ralph Nader and Naders' Raiders will be included.

Consumer Federation of America

The Consumer Federation of America serves as a unifying coalition of consumer organizations at the local, state, regional, national, and international levels. It has at least 196 member organizations representing such constituencies as local, state, and national consumer groups; women's clubs; labor unions; farm groups; cooperatives; and affiliations of senior citizens. It is dedicated to promoting the rights of consumers, has waged campaigns for workable warranties, has tried to reform the Federal Trade Commission, has opposed unfair credit cards, and has insisted upon the creation of an independent consumer agency at the Federal level. *News from CFA,* its periodic bulletin, serves as a clearing house for information on issues, programs, and activities affecting consumers.

Consumers Union

Chartered in February, 1936, Consumers Union (CU) is a tax-exempt nonprofit institution. The founders of this independent testing organization reasoned that Americans needed a magazine to inform them about the quality of the products they bought for the price paid. Previously, a test facility, Consumers Research, was formed in 1929. This group later became Consumers Union.

The first issue of *Consumer Reports* went to 3000 charter subscribers in May, 1936. Early issues informed its readers about the costs and nutritional values of breakfast cereals, claims made for Alka Seltzer, hazards of lead toys, and identified good buys in toilet soaps and tooth brushes.

Advertising agencies and manufacturers had been increasing their pressure on consumers to buy irrationally in 1936 as they do today. Some of the gimmicks still used are promises of instant sex appeal, clothes washed whiter than white, instant energy from processed foods, relief from colds by some over-the-counter drug, or instant good health from certain tonics. In 1936 advertising persuasion cost less than $15 per person. In 1970 advertising expenditures had reached $100 per person in the United States. Even with inflationary effects on the dollar, the expenditures to advertise retail goods and services rose from $1.9 billion in 1936 to $20 billion in 1970. In most instances the consumers were paying for false promises and rarely got product-by-product value comparisons.

Consumers Union seeks to satisify real consumer needs and concerns in six ways. First, Consumers Union calls for safer information or designs and, if needed, government intervention where products are likely to injure or even kill the consumer. Second, it discovers sellers who are downgrading their products or deceiving their consumers with hidden price increases or other gimmicks. Third, it documents and proposes rules where credit practices are designed to extort unreasonable prices and to indenture poverty-level consumers. Fourth, Consumers Union suggests a less costly and more workable system when an industry seems unable to supply the services for which its customers pay. Fifth, it suggests new standards of responsibility when warranties are not assurances of a manufacturer's faith in his products. Sixth, Consumers Union reveals those governmental regulators who cater to the desires of commercial interests instead of fulfilling their legal functions.

Every month more than 4000 letters come to Consumers Union requesting information on products and services in the marketplace. These requests, results of the annual questionnaire sent to 300,000 CU members, surveys by CU's Marketing Information Division, findings of the Survey Research Unit, and other information gathered by the CU staff determine the products or services to be tested. The preliminary test procedures include information on prices in retail stores, availability, and industry marketing practices; product specifications; varieties of the same product; and selection of test methods. If a standard test method has been developed, such as one by the American National Standards Institute or by the National Bureau of Standards, it may be used. Where no standards exists, CU engineers develop their own test methods.

Identification labels are removed from products and code numbers are substituted before tests begin. The testing involves laboratory tests, statistically designed use-panel tests, and controlled-use tests. The laboratory tests determine product's performance and convenience in use, its economy of operation, its safety, and durability. Statistically designed use-panel tests are those actually involving consumers. Controlled-use tests involve experts, professional consultants, and CU's engineers with special expertise. A comprehensive report on the results of the testing is prepared by CU's engineers. The report includes how the tests were conducted, how comparative quality ratings were determined, and special information. The report is distributed to the editorial, library, and marketing departments. The writer for the *Consumer Reports* article develops an outline covering significant findings and suggests the sequence for the final article. Technical, marketing, and editorial personnel discuss, amend, and approve the outline and sequence. As the article is written, into it is woven information from CU marketing and other consulting staff members. After editing, it is recirculated to CU's technical, marketing, library, and editorial departments. Rechecking is done by the marketing department as to models of the product and by the library for accuracy against the engineering report. At every production stage, the article is recirculated for checking by all CU staff concerned. The final article reports why the product was chosen, what meaningful differences were found among tested brands, and how the brands were rated in overall quality. Thus, the consumer can use the report to get more value for his money.

CU's executives, researchers, and engineers have testified at legislative committees and at regulatory agency hearings of the federal government. The organization has brought suit against the Veterans Administration so as to force release of government data on performance of hearing aids purchased by the government. Consumers Union has initiated or supported legal actions and petitions to regulatory agencies to prod them to act on hazardous products and anticonsumer practices (false or deceptive advertising). If regulatory agencies take unsatisfactory action or none at all, readers of Consumer Reports are informed. It has sponsored or participated in national conferences, provided modest financial support to encourage research on consumer problems, served as a resource for educators and community leaders, and provided science writers and broadcasters with summaries of test findings.[4]

Better Business Bureaus

Better Business Bureaus located in the chief business centers throughout the United States aim to protect the businessman and consumer. As nonprofit organizations, these bureaus promote accuracy in advertising, fight frauds, reduce unfair competition, and educate the public and its members. Complaints are solicited, and consumer education is made available. Mobile units may tour areas with low-income families.

Local bureaus are affiliated with the national association which coordinates activities of local bureaus. The national organization handles inquiries and investigates complaints on an interstate basis. It provides services to communities without local bureaus. Local bureaus provide information to inquiries about businesses in that vicinity and receive complaints. The inquiries are answered by factual information given by businesses to questionnaires from the bureaus. A large percentage of the complaints are about mail-order purchases, misleading advertising, mail-order insurance, and quack remedies for weight reduction, arthritis, and nutritional deficiencies. Local bureaus do not handle complaints about medical, legal, and credit bureau charges. Complaints must be in writing and be accompanied by a letter sent to the business. The local bureaus do not recommend or endorse a product.

A resident of a local community may inquire about a business or file a written complaint of fraud about a business, free of charge. The bureau investigates and finds the facts about the business through its own sources or cooperation with other agencies. Officials of the bureau contact executives of the business and urge the executives to correct the complaint, if justified. If the executives take no action, more drastic action may need to be taken. Often the bureau publishes and distributes a bulletin describing the malpractice by the business. Law-enforcement agencies may be involved in the case if the business continues the malpractice. The bureau tries to prevent malpractice among businesses. When fraudulent practices occur, the bureau takes the necessary procedures to eradicate them. Arbitration programs have been established in more than 80 major cities. The threat of arbitration often brings a voluntary settlement.

The Health and Safety Division of the national organization develops cooperative programs with governmental regulatory agencies and health professions. It promotes the concept of voluntary self-regulation as described in Chapter 5. It promotes consumer education of the public and organizations interested in the consumer.

American Medical Association

Five departments or councils of the American Medical Association (AMA) control fraudulent practices to the consumer: Department of Investigation, Department of Health Education, Council on Foods and Nutrition, Council on Physical Medicine, and Council on Drugs. The Department of Investigation (Chapter 1) investigates quacks, medical quackery, patent medicines, medical fads, and pseudomedicine.

The Department of Health Education tries to motivate people to take responsibility for living healthfully and to encourage others to do the same. Three Congresses on the Quality of Life were organized in the belief that "this country possesses the vision, resources, and technology to free people from their social and physical limitations and to help them to achieve a better quality of life." The AMA also believes that health education is the "key to people's ability to make wise use of scientific and social advances."[5]

The Council on Foods and Nutrition investigates all types of food faddism and weight reduction quackery, mentioned in Chapters 1 and 2, in addition to disseminating information and undertaking research on nutrition and dietary habits. "Smart Eating" by the Director of Foods and Nutrition appears each month in *Today's Health*.

The Council on Physical Medicine investigates and reports on non-medical apparatus and devices offered to physicians, hospitals, and the public. The Council on Drugs judges drugs that claim to have therapeutic value. The accepted products are discussed in the *Journal of the American Medical Association*.

American Dental Association

The Council on Dental Therapeutics of the American Dental Association has been evaluating products used in the treatment and prevention of dental diseases since 1930. The first edition of *Accepted Dental Remedies*, which listed and evaluated dental products, appeared in 1934. These dental products include toothpastes, tooth powders, mouthwashes making therapeutic claims in advertising, tooth brushes (manual and electric), and dental floss.

The Association has published many studies about fluoridation of community water supplies. It has supported state and local dental societies and state and local health departments in their community efforts to have voters recognize the values of fluoridation of community water supplies.

American Dietetic Association and American Home Economics Association

Two professional groups that encourage nutrition education programs in schools and colleges are the American Dietetic Association and the American Home Economics Association. Their programs are designed to provide students with an understanding of grades of commodities, standards, and services for consumers. One of the basic purposes of these two groups is to combat food faddism (Chapter 2). Both groups publish a monthly journal and other publications of interest to the consumer.

Other Agencies

Other nongovernmental agencies are the National Association of Consumers, National Consumer-Retailer Council, Good House-keeping Institute and Investigation Service, *Parents' Magazine,* and the following semicommercial groups:

American Institute of Baking
Cereal Institute
Evaporated Milk Association
Florida Citrus Commission
National Board of Fire Underwriters
National Dairy Council
National Livestock and Meat Board
Nutrition Foundation, Inc.
Pharmaceutical Manufacturers Association
Wheat Flour Institute

Some examples of commercial groups are Aetna Life Affiliated Companies, Employers Mutual of Wausau, Equitable Life Assurance Society of the United States, John Hancock Mutual Life Insurance Company, and Metropolitan Life Insurance Company. These groups publish pamphlets and bulletins concerning health insurance and other health information for the consumer. Many food companies, for example, Borden, Carnation Milk, General Mills, H. J. Heinz, Kellogg Company, and Kraft Cheese have distributed literature on nutrition for the consumer. Pharmaceutical companies such as Eli

Lilly, Johnson & Johnson, and Lederle Laboratories have published pamphlets on vaccines, first aid supplies, and over-the-counter drugs. Lever Brothers and Proctor and Gamble have printed materials on dental health products, as well as other health products for the consumer.

Voluntary community health agencies, some mentioned in Chapters 1 and 2, distribute consumer information. Some of these agencies are:

American Cancer Society
American Diabetes Association
American Heart Association
Arthritis Foundation
Epilepsy Foundation of America
Leukemia Society of America, Inc.
Muscular Dystrophy Associations of America, Inc.
National Association of Hearing and Speech Agencies
United Cerebral Palsy Associations, Inc.

The National Association for Mental Health has been aware of the growing number of psychoquacks.

Youth groups such as 4-H clubs and many of our community service organizations provide information for consumers. The National Congress of Parents and Teachers has promoted consumer education in schools. Social clubs, fraternal organizations, labor unions, and patriotic organizations have programs improving the consumer interests of their members.

Ralph Nader and Nader's Raiders

For the past few years, Ralph Nader has been the consumer champion both fervently admired and bitterly hated. In 1966, he authored *Unsafe at Any Speed,* an attack on General Motors' rear-engine *Corvair* and on the whole automotive industry for neglect of safety in auto design. As a result, the Traffic and Motor Safety Act passed in 1966 gave the federal government strong supervisory power over design and manufacture and improved car safety.

Between 1966 and 1970, several legislative acts were passed due to Nader's continuous efforts: Wholesome Poultry Products Act, Wholesome Meat Act, Coal Mine Health and Safety Act, Radiation Control for Health and Safety Act, and Comprehensive Occupational Safety and Health Act. Some of these laws are weak; others are poorly enforced. However, in 1969, Nader's Raiders exposed the inefficiency of the Federal Trade Commission. Since 1970, the FTC has taken many tough actions to police marketing practices and advertising. Nader's most important contribution has been to change the public's attitude toward the products bought, to ask questions of government and corporate officials, and to receive responses for their questions.

Funds for Nader's Raiders and Nader's salary come from donations, fees for speeches, foundation grants, and a direct mail fundraising campaign. Naider's Raiders are a year-round staff of 50 recent college graduates, most of them in their twenties and willing to work at a small yearly salary.

Some of the projects are suits under the Freedom of Information Act to get secrets from the Washington bureaucracy, petitions to force certain governmental regulatory agencies to get tough with industries they are to regulate, investigations of different governmental and nongovernmental agencies with consumer interests, and continuous testimony before Congressional committees investigating toy safety, pension plans, and other consumer affairs. The best of the Nader reports, those on government agencies and policies, are well-documented and unquestionable in facts and conclusions. Some Nader reports question his credibility.

Nader contends that the public can make governmental agencies responsible to public needs. Also, these agencies can operate to satisfy the public's needs at the present time. Nader feels that a *permanent* citizen consumer organization can be established to prevent reoccurrence of past abuses. There is no doubt that Nader is a catalyst of the new consumer consciousness.

REFERENCES

1. Office of the Federal Register, National Archives and Records Service, General Services Administration: United States Government Manual 1973/74. Washington, D.C., July 1973.
2. Dick, C. H.: The way to a consumer's heart. FDA Consumer, 6:10, 1972.
3. Office of the Federal Register, *op. cit.*
4. Continuing need to discover the truth. Consumer Reports, 36:678, 1971.
5. Wesley, W. A.: American Medical Association. School Health Review, 4:2, 1973.

SUPPLEMENTAL READINGS

American Medical Association: Directory of National Voluntary Health Organizations. Chicago, The Association, 1968.

Anderson, C. L.: Community Health, 2nd Edition. St. Louis, C. V. Mosby Company, 1973.

Beyrer, M. K., Nolte, A. E., and Solleder, M. K.: A Directory of Selected References and Resources for Health Instruction. 2nd Edition. Minneapolis, Burgess Publishing Company, 1969.

Biddle, W., and Loureide, J.: Encouraging Community Development. New York, Holt, Rinehart, & Winston, Inc., 1968.

Ginsberg, E., and Ostow, M.: Men, Money, and Medicine. New York, Columbia University Press, 1970.

Hanlon, J. J., and McHose, E.: Design for Health: School and Community. 2nd Edition. Philadelphia, Lea & Febiger, 1971.

Herman, H., and McKay, M. E.: Community Health Services. Washington, D.C., International City Managers' Association, 1968.

Munson, B. E.: Changing Community Dimensions. Columbus, Ohio, Ohio State University Press, 1968.
Smolensky, J., and Haar, F. B.: Principles of Community Health. 3rd Edition. Philadelphia, W. B. Saunders Company, 1972.
Wilson, R. N.: Community Structure and Health Action: A Report on Process Analysis. Washington, D.C., Public Affairs Press, 1968.

Index

260   Index

Devices—*cont'd.*
weight-reducing, 28-30
Diabetes, 31, 104
Diamond Carbon Compound, 9
Dietitian, 42, 229
Diets, arthritis, 45
cancer, 9-10
weight reduction, 26
Zen, 48-49
Digitalis, 26
Director(s), executive, 209
office services, 211
volunteer services, 211
Disability, 123, 136-137
income insurance, 136-137
long-term, 136
short-term, 136
total, 131-132
Disease Control, Center of, 193, 243-244
Diseases, fallacies, 67
periodontal, 17, 18, 19
Diuretics, 26
Doctor, root, 58-60
unethical, 77-79
Double indemnity, 123
Drown Laboratories, mechanical quackery, 22, 83, 104
Drown, Ruth, 22, 104
Drug(s), 177-201
antibiotics, 180
anticancer, 9
brand, 180-181, 194
Bureau of, 180, 186, 241-242
classes, 181, 186-187
compendia, 179-180
data falsification, 182
definition, 177-178
effectiveness, 178-179, 185
generic, 180-181, 194
IND, 181-183
ineffective, 185-186
legislation, 13, 96-100, 103, 106, 178, 185-186, 192, 193
microbiological control, 183-185
NDA, 181, 182-183, 185, 196-197
nursing-home patients, 75
over-the-center (OTC), 186-193
advertising, 93-96
Anacin, 189
Arthritis Pain Formula, 190
Aspirin, 188-191
Bufferin, 189-190
Carter's Little Liver Pills, 187
categories, 186-187
Cope, 190
description, 186
Excedrin, 189-190
Excedrin PM, 190
effectiveness, 187-188
evaluation, 185

Drug(s)—*cont'd.*
hexachlorophene, 192-193
labeling, 186, 187-188
packaging, 191-192
safety, 178-179, 187-188
standards, 187-188
Vanquish 189-190
vitamin E, 14, 51-52, 191
prescription, 193-199
advertising, 93-96
Chloromycetin, 197-199
description, 193-194
label, 194-196
pediatric dose, 196
physician's information, 194-196
pregnancy, 195-196
safety, 178-179
unavailable, 196-197
pricing, 199-200
recalls, 178-179
standards, enforcement, 180-181, 182
federal, 178-179, 181-182, 187-188
industry, 179-180
manufacturing, 182-183
microbiological, 183-185
weight reducing, 26-27
Durham-Humphrey Act, 99-100
Dynamizer, 20

ECONOMIST, Health, 218
Eczema, 14
Educators, information specialist, 214
public health, 213-214
school health, 212-213
Efficacy study, drug, 185
Elective benefits, 123
Electrocardiograph technologist, 232
Electroencephalograph technologist, 232
Electronic Medical Foundation, 21
Electrotherapist, 21
Elixer Sulfanilamide, 98
E-meter, 25
Endodontics, 163
Engineer, biomedical, 227-228
hospital, 227
safety, 228
sanitary, 227
Engrams, 24
Environmental Protection Agency, 47
Epidemiologist, 216
Epilepsy, 31
ERA, 20
Essential Four Food Groups, 37, 48, 50
Estrogen, 26
Evidence of insurability, 123
Examinations, dental, 162
medical, 149, 153
nursing, 167
state board, 153, 162, 167
Excedrin, 189-190

Susto, 62, 64-65
Syphilis, 58

TALISMAN, 55-56
Technologist, blood bank, 232
  cytology, 232
  electrocardiograph, 232
  electroencephalograph, 232-233
  food, 233
  histologic, 232
  medical, 231-233
    nuclear, 232
    radiologic, 233
Teeth, artificial, 19
  dental caries, 17
  dentifrices, 18-19
  fallacies, 66-67
  malocclusion, 17-18
  periodontal diseases, 17
Television advertising, 94
Testing, drugs, 181-183
Therapists, corrective, 235
  educational, 235
  industrial, 236
  inhalation, 236
  manual arts, 235
  music, 235
  occupational, 234-235
  physical, 234
  recreational, 235-236
Thiamin, 38
  RDDA, 41
Thoracic surgery, 156
Thyroxin, 26
Time limit, 125
Today's Health, 95-96, 251
Tonics, cancer, 10
Trademarks, 93, 194
Traiteur, 57
Traiteuse, 57
Tugwell bill, 98
Tulane University School of Medicine, 150
Turtle oil, 12

ULCER, 32-33
Unallocated benefit, 125
United States Department of Agriculture, 47, 239-240
United States Pharmacopeia (USP), 172, 179-180
United States Postal Service, *See also* United States Post Office, 245-246
United States Post Office Department, 43, 95, 101-102
United States Public Health Service, 205, 243-244
  Center for Disease Control, 193, 243-244
  Food and Drug Administration. *See* Food and Drug Administration

U.S. Pub. Health Service—*cont'd.*
  Health Resources Administration, 243
  Health Services Administration, 243
  National Institutes of Health, 244
University of Texas, Medical Branch, Galveston, 150-151
  Nursing School (system-wide), 165-167
Urinalysis, fake, 78
Urology, 156
Utensils, cooking, 50

VACCINES, cancer, 9
Vanquish, 189-190
Vegetables, 69
Verticare, 169
Veterinarian, 224-225
Veterinary Medicine, Bureau of, 242
Vinegar, honey and, 45-46
Virologist, 216
Vitamin(s), fallacies, 69
  fat-soluble, 38-39
    RDDA, 40
  food faddism, 51-52
  water-soluble, 38
    RDDA, 41
Vitamin A, 38
  RDDA, 40
Vitamin B_6, RDDA, 41
Vitamin B_{12}, RDDA, 41
Vitamin C, 38
  faddism, 49, 51
  RDDA, 41, 49
Vitamin D, 38-39
  RDDA, 40
Vitamin E, 191
  cosmetic quackery, 14, 191
  food faddism, 51-52, 191
  RDDA, 40, 191
Voluntary health agencies, 206
  careers, 209, 211, 214
Voluptuizer, 22-23
Voodoo, 56-58
  doctors, 57
  queens, 57
  Southern Louisiana, 57-58

WAITING PERIOD, 125
Waiver, 125
Washes, eye, 16-17
Water, 39-40
  bottled, 50
  sea and ocean, 50
Water-soluble vitamin, 38
Weight reduction, 25-31
  candies, 27-28
  diets, 26
  drugs, 26-27
  fallacies, 69-70
  gadgets, 28-29
  health clubs, 30-31